T0141358

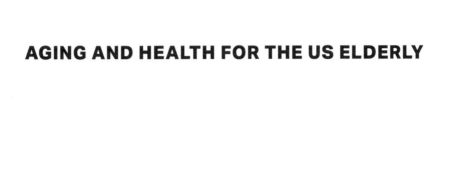

AGING AND HEALTH FOR THE US ELDERLY

AGING AND HEALTH FOR THE US ELDERLY

A Health Primer for Ages 60 to 90 Years

HAROLD L. KENNEDY, MD, MPH, FACC, FAHA

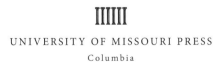

UNIVERSITY OF MISSOURI PRESS
Columbia

Library of Congress Cataloging-in-Publication Data

Names: Kennedy, Harold L., author.
Title: Aging and health for the US elderly : a health primer for ages 60 to
    90 years / by Dr. Harold L. Kennedy.
Description: Columbia : University of Missouri Press, 2021. | Includes
    bibliographical references and index.
Identifiers: LCCN 2021007063 (print) | LCCN 2021007064 (ebook) | ISBN
    9780826222435 (hardcover) | ISBN 9780826274618 (book)
Subjects: LCSH: Older people--Medical care--United States. | Older
    people--Services for--United States. | Older people--Care--United
    States.
Classification: LCC RA564.8 .K44 2021 (print) | LCC RA564.8 (ebook) | DDC
    362.1084/6--dc23
LC record available at https://lccn.loc.gov/2021007063
LC ebook record available at https://lccn.loc.gov/2021007064

∞™ This paper meets the requirements of the
American National Standard for Permanence of Paper
for Printed Library Materials, Z39.48, 1984.

Typefaces: Minion and Aktiv Grotesque

Contents

Illustrations

Figures

....

Tables

Foreword

A nationally renowned cardiologist and public health expert, Dr. Harold Kennedy has been a leader in cardiovascular medicine for decades. In this thoughtful and comprehensive book he dispenses practical and straightforward healthcare advice to those who need it most, Americans aged 60 years and older. In so doing he incorporates instructive medical lessons from U.S. history, such as that of President Franklin Delano Roosevelt's steadily rising blood pressure from the time he took up residence at 1600 Pennsylvania Avenue to the day of his death on April 12, 1945. In another inventive way to reach his readership , Kennedy invokes famous movies such as *Rambo* to illustrate his points.

Above all else, Kennedy emphasizes the importance for all adults to improve their health literacy by forming a clear understanding of the hard evidence that supports the recommendations of leading organizations such as the American Cancer Society, the American Heart Association, and the American College of Cardiology. Dr. Kennedy organizes these important topics with an easy-to-follow "ABC" approach to the prevention and management of cardiovascular disease, certain forms of cancer, heart failure, and the heart rhythm abnormality known as atrial fibrillation.

A: Assessment of Risk – Here Kennedy describes in plain language the lessons learned from important epidemiologic research such as the Framingham Heart Study, which taught us about the traditional modifiable and nonmodifiable risk factors for heart disease and stroke. He also deals squarely with the social determinants of disease and health, those associated with socioeconomic and environmental factors, overlooked but just as important as genetic determinants. In short, one's home zip code is as important as one's genetic code.

A: Antiplatelet/Anticoagulant Therapy – Here Kennedy analyzes the current thinking about how the recommendations supporting the use of aspirin and other antiplatelet agents differ based on the patient's age and whether one has incurred a prior cardiovascular disease event. He also shares his thoughts on when stronger blood thinners known as anticoagulants are indicated in persons with atrial fibrillation.

B: Blood pressure – For many years, the goals for systolic blood pressure control used to be 100 + a person's age. Subsequently, randomized controlled trials and observational data now support the view that all adults and children should aim for a blood pressure of < 130/80 by trying to improve lifestyle habits. For those who cannot succeed through diet and exercise alone, we now have many types of safe and reliable medication from which to choose. In addition, certain classes of these newer blood-pressure medications are specifically indicated to lower the risk of heart failure.

C: Cholesterol – Just as for blood pressure, we now have excellent data that challenges the long-prevailing recommendations by recommending that adults achieve much lower levels of LDL in order to markedly reduce their risk of future cardiovascular events. While statin therapy is the most prescribed cholesterol-lowering agent, there are now several classes of cholesterol-lowering medications with which the reader need be familiar in order to make the best choice.

C: Cigarette/tobacco – complete abstinence from standard combustible cigarettes and electronic cigarettes is an integral part of prevention efforts. For readers who need help breaking their addiction to tobacco products, Kennedy explains the effectiveness of nicotine replacement therapy, which uses new prescription medications such as varenicline or buproprion.

D: Diet/weight – Eating a healthy diet rich in fruits and vegetables and achieving a healthy weight is the cornerstone of one's efforts to lower the risk of cardiovascular disease, cancer, heart failure, and atrial fibrillation

E: Exercise – All Adults should aim for a minimum of 150 minutes of moderate to brisk physical activity a week and preferably > 200 minutes a week.

As you can see, Dr. Kennedy's primer on health will be of great value to all elderly Americans interested in making good decisions about their health and that of their loved ones. I will also be of value to physicians and other healthcare professionals who treat persons in this age range, helping them convey important medical advice.

Roger S. Blumenthal, MD, FACC, FAHA
The Kenneth Jay Pollin Professor of Cardiology
Director, Ciccarone Center for the Prevention of Cardiovascular Disease
Baltimore, MD

AGING AND HEALTH FOR THE US ELDERLY

PART I.

PRIMER OF HEALTH LITERACY

CHAPTER ONE

Introduction to Part I

THIS CONCISE PRIMER of health information is designed as an
optimal health care guide for seniors between the ages of 60 and
90 in the US in the decade of 2020. Seniors find themselves in
the digital age of rapidly advancing medical discoveries which
all too often are difficult to access within a deteriorating system
of optimal health care delivery. Today 617 million people are 65
years or older; by 2050, the number could grow to 1.6 billion
(20% of the world's population), and the population of the "oldest
old" (80 years or greater) could triple to 447 million.[1,2] In the US
currently, 50.9 million are aged 65 years and older, and by 2030,
all baby boomers will be older than 65 years with a projected
population of 73.1 million comprising 20% of the US population.[3] The coronavirus COVID-19 will alter these projections.
As the data are gathered in the coming years, the disease likely
will be found to have amended the number of elderly survivors
worldwide, particularly those over 80 years.

Aging is a major risk factor to health and a defining challenge
for the US and the globe in the twenty-first century. As others
have drawn attention to, "thirty years were added to average life
expectancy in the 20th century, and rather than imagine the
scores of ways we could use these years to improve quality of life,
we tacked them on at the end (of life). Only old age got longer."[4]
It is daunting to realize that as life expectancy increases and
fertility rates decline, most Western countries become "aging

societies" with more people over 65 years than under 15 years of age.[5] The US is currently reaching that point.

Whereas the arc of life is being extended to nearly 100 years (for many, perhaps, more), the prescription for a healthy life is just being defined.[6] As a result, national organizations are launching initiatives now to improve health care systems and health literacy to cope with the increasing burden of aging.[2, 7, 8] The lack of basic health literacy is widespread in the US affecting older adults, racial and ethnic minorities, nonnative English speakers, and people with low income and education levels.[9]

What is basic health literacy? Health literacy represents the ability of an individual to gain access to, understand, and use information in ways that promote and maintain good health for themselves, their families, and their communities.[10] Health literacy consists of three components: the individual, the community in which they live, and the health care (system) that they access.[11] Knowledge of these basic factors extends the well-being of all individuals.

Dependent on multiple personal determinants (i.e family culture, educational status attained, and socio-economic status) many individuals with limited health literacy encounter difficulties in interpreting basic health information such as hospital discharge orders or medication dosage instructions. Seniors, who are the group that utilizes more health care services, have more chronic diseases, and take more medications than any other age group, have been shown to have the lowest health literacy of any age group.[12] In a recent RAND corporation model of predicted health literacy conducted by the United Health Group, "differences in education, language spoken, health behaviors and health system characteristics contribute to significant variation in health literacy across all US counties."[12] Areas where the highest health literacy is identified shows 15% to 27% have limited literacy, and in the lowest identified counties between 36% and 59% have limited health literacy. Addressing projected health literacy in the US potentially could result in 93,000 fewer hospitalizations, 80,000 fewer readmissions, and 820,000 fewer emergency room visits with a potential savings to the Medicare program of $25.4 billion each year.[12]

This primer serves as an introduction to health literacy, offering a perspective on one's individual life cycle, introducing the concept of comorbidities and its importance, and recognizing the medical era in which one has lived and currently lives. Life's uncertainty demands a basic understanding of the US health care system in 2020, and the individual effects of the SARS-coronavirus-2 Pandemic (COVID-19) currently in progress must be discerned even as the author creates this primer.

With that knowledge, this primer offers an idealized pyramid of personal health for the senior citizen from a preventive perspective. As a senior physician, the author has observed that preventive health and medical care, economic stability and peace of mind, and the attainment of personal social and psycho-physiological contentment are essential for personal health. The author, from experience and hindsight, is committed to following evidenced-based medicine from randomized clinical trials to evaluate risk versus benefit for an individual patient.[13] The author's goal is to align remaining life span with existing health knowledge, to understand and compress existing morbidities, and to direct preventive and surveillance actions to sustain quality of life with functionality to the end of life.

This primer is only an initial step in health literacy, because even as the author reports this information considerable change in the US health system is occurring and can be increasingly anticipated to occur within the next five years.[5, 6] Geopolitical and economic forces at work in the US election year of 2020 and the occurrence of the COVID-19 pandemic with its demands on the population being served undoubtedly will shape the US health care system. Even in the health arena the coronavirus COVID-19 is presenting global challenges to many international economies not only with regards to their public health sector, but also the secondary economic effects on their population resulting from diminished economic activity. How this global pandemic will evolve is an open question, but substantial challenges and uncertainty in the US will persist in this age of digital rapid communication. Having been trained in epidemiology (Johns Hopkins School of Public Health) as well as cardiology and internal medicine, the author seeks to report these events as they occur.

Whether this primer delivers "holistic care" may be debatable, but the guidance provided in this primer is derived from astute professional observations of patients who lived in both the twentieth and the twenty-first centuries. The multidimensional nature of human biology and the effects of the world around us (the environment, lifestyle, and social determinants of disease) all play a role in individual aging and health outcomes. The enclosed advice is supported by scientific evidence when it exists as shown in the references, and by the author's more than sixty years of professional experience. This primer is not a "magic bullet" to solve all the problems faced by the elderly. But its perspective and established data, sometimes supported by vignette patient experiences encountered by the author, should prove to be a valuable foundation of elderly health literacy in the US to its readers.

CHAPTER TWO

Life's Cycle

WHEREAS THE POPULAR view of life sometimes is seen as a "roller coaster with many ups and downs," a physician must understand life as a continual path with a beginning and an end. As shown in Figure 1, most persons in the US can expect a maximal arc of a life span of 100 years. The most current data of the US population (2010 US Census of 308.7 million persons) show, however, that 87% attained age 65, 7% attained age 75, 4.2% attained age 85, and only 1.7% live beyond 85 years of life.[14] Within that life span, there are **non-adaptive factors** which the individual has no control over (e.g., their genetic inheritance from their parents), and there are **adaptive factors** (e.g., lifestyle decisions they make about diet and activities). However, the range of lifestyle choices may not be so broad when a person must conform to a specific environment, maintain employment under less than optimal circumstances, or remain in a specific culture. Humans impose these adaptive factors in various ways to achieve specific goals or passions in their individual lives. Nevertheless, adaptive and non-adaptive factors affect the ongoing process of aging and the development of comorbidities that are in progress during the life cycle.

Figure 1 illustrates the stages of life from the author's perspective as a preventive medicine physician. Humans evolve and progress from an *Early Origin* period, to a *Formative* educational period, and then a *Transitional* period before becoming *Elderly*. US culture in the twenty-first century (particularly from adverse

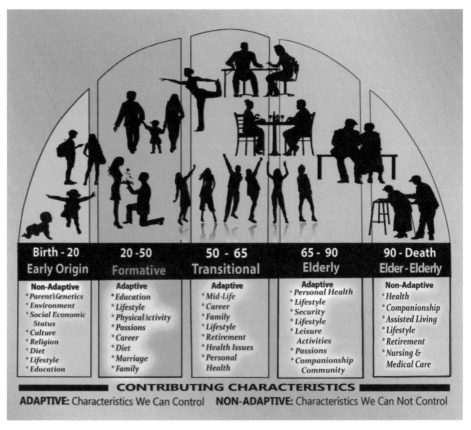

FIGURE 1. Health Arc of change during an aging lifespan.

economic events) has increasingly merged the *Transitional* period of life into the *Elderly* stage, to be followed by the *Elder-elderly* stage.

As shown in Figure 1, the non-adaptive *early origin* period of our lives in the US often extends 18 to 22 years. We are born to parents whose genetics bring us a risk of their health maladies or perhaps a promise of a "long life" from knowledge of their immediate ancestors' health. But the parents' social-economic status at the time may have imposed personal health risks on each of us individuals through their access (or lack of) to medical services and the state of their medical knowledge. Our parents' choice of environment, culture, and religion influences our early lives. Imagine being born into the author's era of 1940. Tobacco cigarette smoking was the rage of the day, and it was portrayed as glamorous, hip and "in" at all socioeconomic levels. Smoking undoubtedly affected some individuals as secondary smoke in some households, whereas perhaps others began smoking as teenagers on a primary basis because of its apparent acceptability. Recent data have shown that adopting cigarette smoking at an early age (<15 years) exerts the highest risk (three to five times) of premature death (before 75 years) from cardiovascular disease.[15] Of course, there were individual variations on this theme. Perhaps one lived in a city with smog or factories with particulate matter in the air, or visited public places with high smoke content (restaurants and some public buildings). On the other hand, it is possible that family culture and religion protected one on a primary basis, but the lack of medical knowledge and the cultural support for smoking nonetheless exposed many to silent lung injury.

Let us reflect on knowledge gained during the current medical era. As shown in Figure 2, the amount of pre-existing lung injury, as measured by a simple pulmonary function study, can predict a shortened life span.[16] Cigarette smoking and air particulate matter have for several decades been linked to adenocarcinoma of the lung, chronic obstructive lung disease, and more recently to the increasing prevalence and incidence of chronic lung disease and asthma in children and young adults.[17, 18] Nonetheless, most of us had no control over the secondary smoke we encountered or the smog/air particulate matter in our environment which recently has been reported globally to account for a shortening of life by roughly 2.9 years and increased prevalence of atrial fibrillation.[19, 20] We were engaged in American society acquiring education and skills that provided little free time to reflect upon our health and well-being. Be cognizant however, that while this aging process was occurring even during childhood

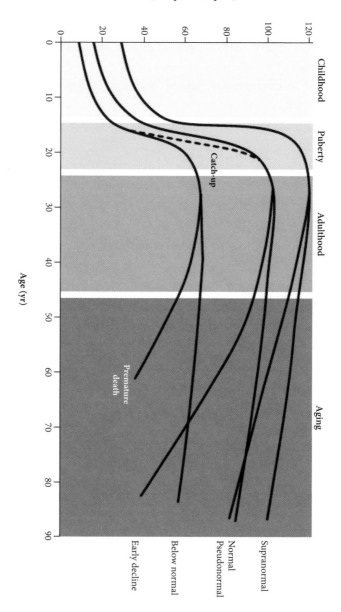

FIGURE 2. Lung-function trajectories from birth to death. Adapted from Augusti A, et al.[16]

each of us was at risk of carrying some silent or known injury (comorbidity) forward that would impact the rest of his/her life. Nevertheless, these predominantly non-adaptive factors have also shaped our individual health in shaping our earliest attitudes toward diet, exercise, lifestyle, and medical education.

In the adaptive *formative life* period of 20 to 50 years of age, most individuals place their individual health below other priorities in the current medical era (Figure 1). If they are fortunate enough to not have inherited or encountered a serious disability or disease (the vast majority), they typically focus on seeking to achieve a career or skills for sustenance, following a creative passion, or seeking a marriage and family with a desire for an improved individual lifestyle. This has been the usual template of American life. That left limited time for reflection on ongoing personal aging and possible health comorbidities. Nevertheless, as education, work career, marriage and children seem to absorb the mainstream of life until age 50, hopefully individuals have enjoyed access to medical care during this time to limit chronic comorbidities. Sometime around the age of 50 years, most people begin to acknowledge that they are entering the declining years of life. Many persons in the current elderly population have not reflected upon their inherited disorders, transient injuries, and silent medical comorbidities. These sources of illness, encountered by every individual in a lifespan whether recognized or not (i.e., they are silent), are the comorbidities of each person's health. This pattern has been true for individuals in both the twentieth and twenty-first centuries.

The adaptive *transitional life* period occurs sometime after age 50 years, when the individual becomes conscious and realizes that he/she is in the second half of life. Not everyone may undergo a "mid-life crisis," but American society makes it hard to ignore retirement planning, social security, Medicare, and leaving the workforce at age 65 to 67 years; these transitions sustain the economics of today's society. An integral part of American society and the economic interests associated with it is preparing for future economic stress and anxiety by investing in a 401(k) and acting on other retirement suggestions during our *formative* lives. However, these strategies often did not work as shown by substantial current data.[21] In today's society, regrettably, less than half the adult population of America has addressed the economic and health concerns associated with aging. Fortunately, the advances of the modern medical era have allowed many persons to extend their work life to 70 years and beyond. It is during this period of life when the specter of comorbidities or "underlying conditions" appears, and one begins to encounter unexpected illness, disabilities, and a potential early death.

This is a time in life when many individuals reflect upon their life choices and experiences and reassess their goals, wishes, and personal outcomes. This reflection and their own experience kindle a concern for individual health adaptation for the vast majority of individuals. The most popular current concern is focused on access to health services and care in the early twenty-first century. Some people become interested in preventive medical knowledge. Some seek to choose a healthier lifestyle. Others weigh climate change with its effects upon their health and pursue optimal environmental conditions. Many are trying to prepare for the *elderly* period of life. Hopefully, with the current COVID-19 pandemic knowledge of the importance of basic preventive health habits (including the need for vaccines) will be clearly understood and practiced in their daily lives. Unfortunately, many elderly individuals are already carrying comorbidities, which will affect their future health and determine their risk during the ongoing pandemic.

The *elderly* life period occurs from 65 to 90 years. It may be adaptive or non-adaptive depending on the success or lack of success, and comorbidities the individual brings to it. Currently, many Americans who have encountered favorable circumstances throughout life seek travel and leisure activities with good health. In contrast, some of the population with health challenges may spend up to approximately one-third of their day on health and related issues with the quality of their life affected by their comorbidities and any new emerging threats from aging which occur concomitantly. During this period of life many individuals' perspectives and priorities change with health and wellness becoming more important, because of the limited number of years remaining. The elderly population confronts a pyramid of concerns and worries concerning health (discussed below). As currently recognized, medical advances in the twentieth century added thirty years to our average life expectancy, and the majority of those years prolonged the period of old age. This has resulted in anxieties ("I hope I do not get dementia.") or worried questions ("Will I outlive my money?").[4] Finally, for the fortunate few who survive and are in the category of the *elder-elderly* (greater than 85 to 90 years), conditions imposed by frailty, comorbidities, and ongoing health issues can lead to a period of non-adaptive lifestyle with fewer choices or less control in a nursing or assisted living facility. The minority of elder-elderly who remain adaptive from the success of their lives and sustained health continue pursuing their passions and interests to the end of their lives.

The author has observed and participated in every social stratum of American life, having rendered care to the poorest of our society, as well as to the wealthy living in great luxury, and having observed health patterns from East to West coast, and from North to South geographically in the US. This experience must be placed within the perspective of the current medical era in 2020, and hopefully a positive perspective will be conveyed to and adopted by the reader.

CHAPTER THREE

Comorbidities

COMORBIDITIES, AS DEFINED by Merriam Webster dictionary, denotes a condition "existing simultaneously with and usually independently of another medical condition." This definition, however, does not resonate in our consciousness until we consider how, what, and when a silent asymptomatic condition impacts us during our life cycle. Table 1 lists some frequent silent (asymptomatic) comorbidities and known (conscious) comorbidities all humans face as they navigate the years of their lives. The sage financier of our times, Warren Buffet, has given advice to millennials to regard their health as they would a "prized car," something they get only once in a lifetime.[22] "You're probably going to read the owner's manual four times before you drive it; you're going to keep it in the garage, protect it at all times, change the oil twice as often as necessary," said Buffett. "If there's the least little bit of rust, you're going to get that fixed immediately so it doesn't spread—because you know it has to last you as long as you live." He went on to add: "You have only one mind and one body for the rest of your life. . . . If you aren't taking care of them when you're young, it's like leaving that car out in hailstorms and letting rust eat away at it. If you don't take care of your mind and body now, by the time you're 40 or 50, you'll be like a car that can't go anywhere."[22]

It is daunting to realize how seemingly minor events in life impact our daily health when we are elderly. To illustrate this

TABLE 1. Silent and known comorbidities.

Silent Comorbidities
Air particle matter damage (future lung chronic changes)
Secondary smoke (future COPD, bronchitis and lung cancer)
Hypertension (high blood pressure - future heart disease and stroke)
Hyperlipidemia (high cholesterol or triglycerides leads to atherosclerosis)
Small oral airway leading to snoring and various Sleep Apnea (future hypertension and atrial fibrillation)
Lack of exercise or sedentary activity (future decreased immunity)
Silent and unrecognized vascular events (heart attacks, emboli and inflammation).
Residual bacterial (Tuberculosis) or viral (Parkinson's Disease) illness

Known Comorbidities Often Sustained by the Patient
History of "bad colds" or pneumonia
Sport injuries (e.g. concussions, repeated trauma to joints, broken bones, knee and hip wear and tear, etc.)
Automobile accidents with delayed neck or back injuries
History of hepatitis or infectious mononucleosis
Vaping lung injury
Diabetes m, adult type
Discovered metabolic risk factors
Lack of exercise

point, here is a vignette of an actual patient with a sport injury comorbidity:

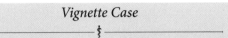

Vignette Case

The patient at the age of 17 years described how during his youth to impress his peers, he undertook a substantial ski jump (30 meters) without much skill or knowledge. It resulted in a major left medial ankle sprain for which he did not receive proper treatment. The patient had no access to medical care, and during this era (the 1950s), there were no air casts or similar splints as utilized today. This resulted in the onset of a gradual pes planus (flat arch) of the left foot, which subsequently affected the knee tilt of that inferior extremity. The patient then sustained a right anterior cruciate ligament injury during the sport of judo at age 42 years. This injury was repaired by open knee surgery in 1980. Subsequently, at age 46 years, the patient became aware of marked pes planus in both feet and had to resort to orthotics in all shoes to relieve pain created at both arches. Over the years, this malady gradually became more and more pronounced. At age 75 years, while lifting a fifty-pound bag of yard seed, the patient experienced severe acute lower back pain. He was unaware of how the orthopedic changes of his lower extremities had conditioned him to have substantial changes in his lumbosacral spine. Orthopedic and MRI examination of his lower back revealed a compression fracture at the L5-S1 interspace, and the patient now experiences low back pain (scale of 1 to 2 out of 10) every morning which gradually improves with movement or tai chi exercises. He treats this malady currently at age 80 years with intermittent anti-inflammatory medications, and to date has declined any surgical interventions.

Of a more serious nature are the insidious silent comorbidities that impact medical diseases such as heart disease, stroke, and cancer. In the current medical community, these are referred to as **health risk factors**. That was not the case for the existing medical knowledge in the 1940s and 1950s when the Framingham Heart Study project began in Framingham, Massachusetts.[23] At that time, the threat of heart attacks and sudden death were prevalent in North America. The Framingham Heart Study is a long-term, cardiovascular cohort (group of persons with specific factors in a specific geographic location) study of residents of the city of Framingham, Massachusetts. The study began in 1948 with 5,209 adult subjects and is now on its third generation of participants. Prior to the study almost nothing was known about the epidemiology of hypertensive or arteriosclerotic cardiovascular disease. Much of the now-common knowledge concerning heart disease and high blood pressure, such as the effects of diet, exercise, and common medications such as aspirin, are based on this longitudinal study. It is a project of the National Heart, Lung and Blood Institute, in collaboration with (since 1971) Boston University.[23, 24] Health professionals from the hospitals and universities of Boston staff the project.

This study identified the role of blood cholesterol and hyperlipidemia (high blood lipids) in the occurrence of heart attacks and led to a medical paradigm shift; obtaining fasting blood studies is a routine measurement in today's normal physical examination. This was the beginning of the identification of risk factors in predicting an association or outcome to a specific disease. Framingham study observations on the importance of those factors coupled with the importance of hypertension resulted in the identification of key elements of the arteriosclerotic process leading to thrombotic occlusion of the coronary arteries now known to be the genesis of myocardial infarctions or heart attacks.[25] The medical experts of the last century had previously regarded the process well into the 1960s and 1970s as "rust in our pipes," and today we know that a universe of knowledge and molecular factors reside in the walls of blood vessels.[25] Today's efforts at reducing the global burden of cardiovascular disease are clearly focused on alteration of lifestyle risk factors (poor diet, little exercise, sedentary activity, and tobacco use), and detection and treatment of hypertension, cholesterol lowering, and antithrombotic therapy.[26, 27] Nevertheless, many persons without knowledge of their heritable risk factors due to a lack of health literacy or access to medical care have carried hypertension and hyperlipidemia as silent comorbidities through a major portion of their adulthood until a social requirement (e.g., an insurance examination) leads to the serendipitous discovery of their malady. The most recent data indicate that the cardiovascular disease burden attributable to modifiable risk factors continues to increase globally.[27]

As the World Health Organization seeks to reduce noncommunicable diseases of the four major causes of mortality (cardiovascular disease, cancer, diabetes mellitus, and chronic respiratory disease) by 25% by 2025, health related behaviors of diet, tobacco use, alcohol consumption, and reduced physical activity currently loom large as risk factor targets.[26, 27, 28] Unfortunately, many of our elderly population have already experienced these silent comorbidities during their life cycle and have carried such comorbidities into the *transition phase* and *elderly* phase of their lives (Figures 1 and 3 on pages 10 and 23). They have belatedly discovered that their risk of a variety of adverse medical and surgical outcomes are determined by the individual status of their pulmonary, cardiovascular, and renal (kidney) function. As shown in Figure 3, these comorbidities can occur without symptoms in a variable manner, but ultimately can affect every individual in the course of their life cycle. Unfortunately, these comorbidities ("underlying conditions") were the dominant factors accounting for 90% of all deaths during the first quarter of the COVID-19 pandemic in the US.

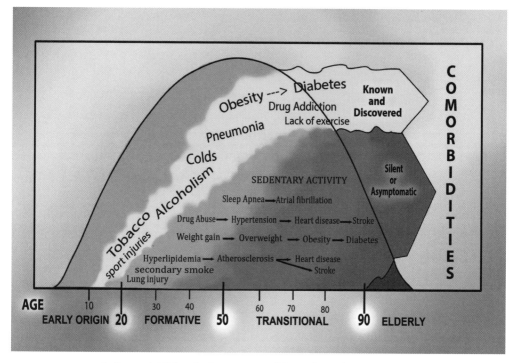

FIGURE 3. Comorbidities during an aging life cycle as they appear during non-adaptive and adaptive periods of life.

Vignette Case

⸙

A 60-year-old man had presented to the author at age 40, and at that time was found to have a renal cell cancer for which he underwent laparoscopic surgery and a partial resection of the kidney. During that hospitalization the patient was discovered to have health risk factors of an elevated cholesterol, hypertension, metabolic syndrome, truncal obesity and a three-packs-per-day cigarette addiction. Family history revealed both parents were heavy smokers, and the father died of hypertension, hyperlipidemia and a suspected subdural (head) blood clot secondary to a fall. Over the course of the twenty years since his last visit the patient had continued to smoke and did not adhere to the medical regimen

22

prescribed for hypertension or hyperlipidemia. He now presents for evaluation of atrial fibrillation.

The patient's wife explains that the patient has insomnia and was observed during January 2020 to have apneic episodes during sleep. They have slept in different rooms for several years because the patient was known to snore loudly. When the patient awoke suddenly with rapid heart beating, he did not feel well, and noted his pulse at 125 to 150 bpm. Alarmed, they went to a private clinic where an electrocardiogram revealed atrial fibrillation. Subsequently, after one day of hospitalization he was started on anticoagulant and advised to see a cardiologist for further therapy. The patient refused and signed out against medical advice. Subsequently in February 2020 during a ski vacation at 1600 meters with his family, the patient awoke short of breath, fatigued, extremely weak, and with rapid heart beating. Emergency medical evaluation disclosed an oxygen level of 90% (SPO2) and sinus heart rhythm. He was advised to return to normal sea level elevations and seek medical evaluation follow up.

Evaluation disclosed that the patient indeed was found to have continued hypertension, hyperlipidemia, and now was morbidly obese (BMI 36). These conditions, coupled with his continued smoking of two and a half packs of cigarettes a day, brought about the onset of atrial fibrillation; the silent comorbidity of increasing obesity with its development of Obstructive Sleep Apnea was a potent stimulus to hypertension and atrial arrhythmias. A sleep study revealed that the patient sustained more than thirty-eight breathing interruptions every hour (AHI i.e., apnea hypopnea index) with oxygen desaturations throughout the night of more than two hours of desaturation below 90%. His "insomnia" was in fact due to obstructive sleep apnea secondary to obesity, and rather than seeking a cardiology procedure for atrial fibrillation alone, he required continuous positive airway pressure (CPAP) through a mask for his obstructive sleep apnea. Although, this patient had known underlying conditions, he also had silent comorbidities. During his evaluation, he was also found to have electrocardiogram evidence suggesting coronary artery disease and evaluation found evidence of peripheral artery disease with occlusion of an artery in a peripheral vessel of the neck. This case was instructive because it revealed both known and silent comorbidities.

CHAPTER FOUR

Medical Eras

The Years 1930 to 1960

EVERY PERSON IS born into a particular medical era. For individuals born in the eras from the 1930s to the 1960s medical knowledge advanced dramatically, adding approximately 30 years to their lifespans. Although recent attention has been drawn to the decrease in life expectancy in the US during the past few years due to opioid overdoses, alcoholism, and suicide,[29] immense changes occurred not only in medical knowledge but also in society in general. Recent evidence shows that socioeconomic status and geography contributed to life expectancy. The difference in life expectancy for the poorest and the wealthiest people in the US was fifteen years, and those living in the South or Midwest were not as likely to live as long as those living in other parts of the country.[30] Since social attitudes toward health, access to health, literacy, environment, and economic conditions all influenced the non-adaptive stage of our early lives, we must reflect on those factors that have affected many of us even today.

The American depression era of the 1930s taught many of us through our parents "that we must eat everything on our plates." Many patients recount stories of how they had to sit at the table until everything was consumed, or they would be fed it the next day. Those early lessons may have contributed to many persons continuing to consume over-abundant meals that were suitable for physical workers of the past but not needed by the industrialized or digital worker of today. The hearty meals of the past are served in many American diners today. This "depression training" undoubtedly has had an undesired effect on many individuals, who continue eating habits into obesity. Increasing obesity and the secondary diabetes adult type resulting from it, serve as an excellent example of how societal events have affected our individual health.

Similarly, in the early twentieth century, the medical system was characterized by general practitioners who practiced alone. In the Midwestern and Western US the "macho pioneer spirit" led many people to claim to "never need a doctor," and bad colds and stomach aches were often ignored. Since hospitals were reserved for the "really bad" things, many silent or unrecognized comorbidities were sustained and now affect those elderly of today. Of course, a lack of medical knowledge and/or progress also contributed to this problem. Based on what is known today, a group of "well appearing" community-dwelling elderly individuals, who experienced unknown heart attacks (myocardial infarctions detected by MRI) had higher rates of death, repeat heart attacks, and heart failure than normal persons without any myocardial infarction at 10-years follow up (Figure 4).[31, 32] This was especially true in the elderly where unrecognized heart attacks are more common than recognized heart attacks.[31, 32] Note on the graphic that after a period of no symptoms, the unknown heart attack victim's mortality rate caught up quickly to persons who had knowledge of their past heart attack (Figure 4). Moreover, today we know that 40% to 50% of persons who die suddenly without a history of heart disease are found at autopsy to have evidence of a silent or unrecognized myocardial infarction.[33, 34]

Similarly, the importance of hypertension, which is now determined to be the single most important health risk factor that affects the most global deaths, was underappreciated in the 1940s and 1950s as evidenced by the death of Franklin D. Roosevelt (Figure 5).[35]

26

All-cause mortality

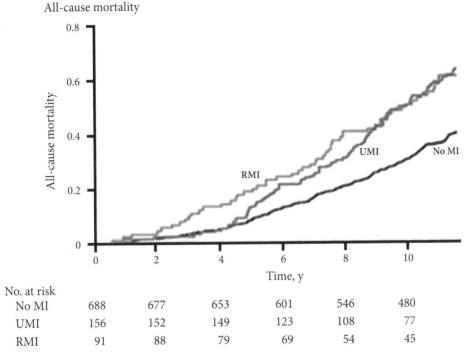

No. at risk						
No MI	688	677	653	601	546	480
UMI	156	152	149	123	108	77
RMI	91	88	79	69	54	45

FIGURE 4. All-cause mortality. RMI, recognized myocardial infarction; UMI, unrecognized myocardial infarction; No MI, normal persons.
Adapted from Acharya T, et al.[31]

Vignette: That Day 75 Years Ago

⚶

"The headlines of April 13, 1945, stunned the nation and the world. Franklin D. Roosevelt, 32nd president of the United States, had died in Warm Springs, Georgia, the day before. Presumably, he had been in excellent health, there was no indication of imminent danger, and as Admiral Ross McIntire, the president's personal physician, asserted, the cerebral hemorrhage 'came out of the clear sky.' Steve Early, press secretary for the White House, stated officially that 'the President was given a thorough examination by seven or eight physicians, including some of the most eminent in the country, and was pronounced organically sound in every way.'"[35]

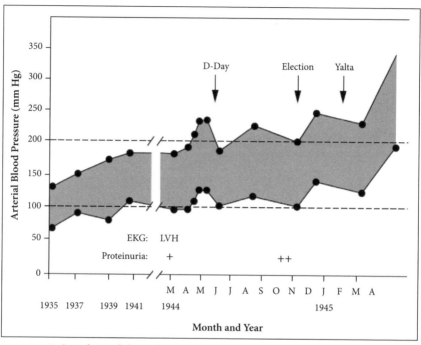

FIGURE 5. Systolic and diastolic arterial pressure of Franklin D. Roosevelt from 1935 to his death on April 12, 1945. EKG, electrocardiogram; LVH, left ventricular hypertrophy. Adapted from Messerli FH[35]

At the time many physicians had adopted the belief that normal blood pressure was expected to be related to the age of the patient. The formula most commonly utilized and printed in many medical texts was the patient's age + 120/80 = blood pressure. As late as 1945, hypertension was not considered a disease of major consequence. It was still viewed by the majority of physicians as "essential" to force blood through sclerotic arteries to the body.[35] It was not until the first successful antihypertensive agents were introduced in the early 1950s, and the studies that followed, that it became clear that treatment led to a substantial reduction in mortality.[36] Pause for a moment to reflect upon the most recent knowledge that the age of onset of hypertension is valuable information, and perhaps must be recognized as a risk factor in itself affecting mortality, cardiovascular disease, and stroke.[37] In those persons who sustain the onset of hypertension before the age of 45 years, the risk of these outcomes is increased 2.0-fold as compared to the patient who becomes hypertensive after age 65.[37] Current medical progress has shown physicians that ambulatory blood pressure measurements provide a better estimate of an individual's cardiovascular disease risk than clinic blood pressures, and both high 24 hour and "masked" asleep blood pressure measurements are associated with an increased risk for all-cause mortality and cardiovascular disease (even after accounting for clinic blood pressure measurements).[38] Unfortunately, false medical assumptions in an earlier era and limited medical knowledge may have affected many persons still alive in today's society.

The Years 1960 to 2020

The author's individual knowledge and medical experiences encompass the time period between 1940 and 2020 (Figure 6). When the author graduated from medical school in the 1960s, it was commonly believed that medical knowledge would change every ten years; it is currently recognized that in today's digital age, fundamental guideline therapies can change within one to two years. Similarly, medical knowledge, which was initially based on symptoms and signs of disease, evolved with studies of cases and then groups of cases. This stage of medical progress was then complemented with comparison to control groups, and subsequently biostatistics evolved and led to the emergence of the randomized control clinical trial. Clearly, today the randomized control clinical trial is the gold standard for establishing the proven benefit of patient therapies, and it is the foundation of evidence-based medicine and clinical medicine (Figure 6).[13, 39] These rapid changes are emerging not only from medical discoveries as occurred in years past, but the application of such discoveries is facilitated by ongoing global randomized clinical trials, large databases of multiple clinical measurements, social

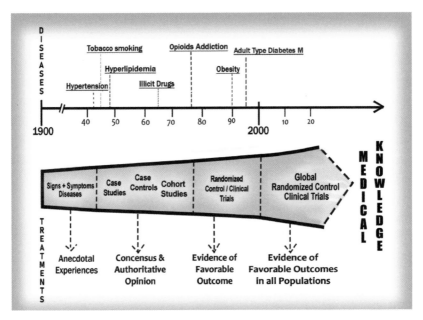

FIGURE 6. Seminal medical discoveries and progress of medical methods from 1940s to 2020.

media dissemination of findings, and intercontinental cooperation in the collection of patient data. The recent employment of artificial intelligence networks to enhance efficiency and interpretation of such data is currently undergoing innovation in today's medical arena.[13]

Figure 7 discloses some of the many seminal discoveries of medical diseases and therapies in the field of cardiovascular medicine during the past eighty years. Obviously, the elderly patients of today can be thankful for the medical progress which has occurred during their lifetime. Although they can regret the comorbidities they may have sustained and carried to their elder status, they can be grateful for the many positive modalities (e.g., coronary artery stents), which exist to provide improved quality of life and an extended lifespan in the current generation. These advances contributed not only to new diagnostic modalities and therapies for signs and symptoms of disease, but proactively contributed to the genesis of identifying "risk factors" in advance of disease onset. Risk assessment of each individual person through investigation of blood studies and noninvasive diagnostic tests (i.e electrocardiogram, echocardiogram, CT and MRI imaging studies) have provided biomarkers (specific factors) that indicate existing health risk to that individual at the time of examination. This change in medical care goals of not only diagnosing and treating medical disease but assessing risk has occurred by marked medical progress in the past forty years. This is discussed more fully below in the "Elderly Health Pyramid" where the prevention, surveillance, and wellness discussion guides the elder to adopt health prevention, personal surveillance, and to make healthful social, environmental, and lifestyle choices. This personal insight and health literacy shared with their caregivers, children, and grandchildren may prove in the long-term to be the most beneficial public health policy of the current era.

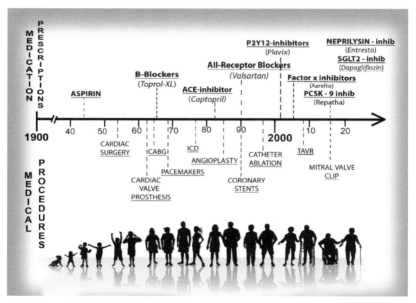

FIGURE 7. Cardiovascular therapeutic progress during the 20th and 21st centuries.

CHAPTER FIVE

The US Health Care System in 2020

WITH SOME RELUCTANCE, the author must indicate to the elderly reader the pitfalls that are currently encountered in the US and its health care system. Political events in 2020, influenced by the COVID-19 pandemic, will define the trajectory of health care in the US in 2021. But for the sake of health literacy, the elderly population should have a basic history of the health care system which developed during their lifetime. During the past twenty to thirty years, accountable care organizations (ACO) have emerged within the US health care arena. These **accountable care organizations** are associations of hospitals, healthcare providers, and insurers in which all parties voluntarily assume financial and medical responsibility for Medicare patients and Medicaid patients. Medicare was created in 1965, because elderly persons over 65 years at the time found it virtually impossible to obtain private health insurance.[40] Many insurance companies avoided insuring the elderly, or when pre-existing medical conditions were identified, they denied coverage or increased rates substantially. Medicare brought the US government into the health equation to guarantee that the elderly could obtain health care services at a reasonable cost. Initially these services were based on a "fee for service" model; that is, all tests and services were paid by the US government at a rate that was set generally lower than that paid by health insurance companies. When Medicare was initiated in 1965, providers resisted what they regarded as lower reimbursement for decades, but the inevitable growth of the elderly population eroded that resistance. By the 1990s, concern for Medicare costs and ongoing funding of the program loomed large in society's medical and political future.[41] Nevertheless, various economic interests, aided by national political lobbying from the pharmaceutical and insurance industry, maintained a fee-for-service model of government reimbursement with overall increasing national medical costs until the introduction of the Affordable Care Act (ACA politically referred to as Obamacare) in 2010.[42] The ACA sought to provide health care insurance to a large group of the uninsured population with protections for those with pre-existing disease conditions. The law also began an effort to base Medicare reimbursement and payments on the provision of favorable outcomes for patients, as determined by evidence-based practices and outcomes.[42] This transition of reimbursement to health care systems for evidence of favorable patient outcomes in return for maximum reimbursement is currently referred to in the industry as "value-based care." This transition to reimbursement for positive clinical outcomes has only emerged during the past decade, and existing today is a mixture of reimbursement of both fee-for-service and outcome measurement goals. The transition is currently ongoing and was the source of substantial stakeholder contention, lobbying, and political attention within the US in 2020. Whereas there are many positive as well as negative aspects of ACO organizations, which are under pressure to demonstrate favorable patient outcomes to obtain maximal Medicare reimbursement, change in their organization of delivering health care has brought some concerns which the author judges to affect the elderly specifically. These concerns include (1) the establishment within the hospital of "hospitalists," (2) the presence of "urgent care" centers within the community, and (3) more recently, point-of-care clinics in pharmacies. It is essential that we review potential pitfalls of these changes with an open mind.

Initially the "hospitalists" were intended to provide a higher level of physician expertise with knowledge of multiple medical fields within the hospital environment. They were envisioned to work in concert with local primary care physicians stationed outside the hospital. The danger of lack of continuity of care was recognized early in the process, but health care systems insisted that the promise of the newly embraced electronic medical records system would overcome the danger of a lack of continuity of care and would lead to cost savings and better medical care. That idealized concept within the author's experience has been achieved in less than 30% to 40% of all health care systems, particularly in local community hospital systems. Between 2000 and 2020, various health care systems changed these policies, limiting the primary care physician's ability to order many hospital tests, and regretfully, many electronic medical record systems were slowly or incompletely developed. We must realize that the traditional model of "continuity of care" (i.e., one doctor responsible for a patient's history, examinations, and medical care) has now, most commonly, become a thing of the past within ACOs. It has been usurped by a system of multiple "specialists" and an electronic medical record system under continuous development and often lacking important information on a specific patient.

Further policies were enacted that limited both primary care and hospital clinical visiting times to fifteen- or twenty-minute encounters, and that encounter time more recently must be reported by the clinicians to the health care system. This "time crunch" all too often does not leave a clinician adequate time to gain a thorough understanding of the history and comorbidities of the elderly patient before addressing his or her concern during a new visit. Whereas the system may work well for the younger patient who has no demonstrated comorbidities, it fails to disclose many important issues that may exist in the elderly patient before their new or current problem visit. If the promised medical electronic record system is not fully developed to correctly integrate past and current data, the brief visit can lead to flawed judgments and adverse outcomes.

Stop and imagine the difficulties that arise because of restrictions imposed by COVID-19 and the increasing promulgation by ACOs of the "telehealth" visit response now emerging in the marketplace.

Because the twenty-first-century Cures Act ensures patient access to electronic health records, recent studies have documented the seriousness of these developments.[43] A survey study of 22,000 patients at three US health care centers with seventy-nine academic and community care practices found errors in 20% of their records with 40% of the errors being serious and very serious.[43] The most common profoundly serious errors (9.9%) were in medical diagnosis, patient history, and medications and allergies. Since an estimated twelve million Americans experience diagnostic error annually, this is not an additional compounding error to be taken lightly.[43, 44] Less than half of hospitals have an electronic health record portal for long-term care facilities to access hospital information, send information electronically to long-term care facilities, or receive training for adults/caregivers on their patient portal.[43]

These developments have led increasingly during the last twenty years to more "concierge medicine" within the US, which is the paying of a fee by individual patients usually on an annual basis to have special access to a clinician who provides them easier access and adequate time for examinations.[45] Notwithstanding the advantages of this model, concierge medicine has evolved into a lifestyle wellness role with an increased emphasis on primary prevention.[46] Obviously, the patient must have the personal resources to afford this avenue of health care. Although no large-scale study of the number older people who use concierge medicine exists, it is suspected that in 2020 less than 5% of the elderly population took advantage of this kind of health care.

In addition to these changes, during the last few years, "urgent care" centers have emerged and been strategically placed and disseminated within local communities by the ACO health care systems.[47] These centers offer the promise of shorter waiting times, convenience of access, and avoidance of long wait times while bringing about lower cost to the health care system and patient.[47] Currently more than 10,000 of these centers exist across the US, and many of these facilities are adequately staffed with modern equipment and testing. But notably they are increasingly being managed by non-physicians (allied health professionals, nurse practitioners, etc.) either for cost-saving reasons or the inability to recruit physicians to this primary care field. Disturbingly, several states have introduced legislation that non-physician providers can work without the supervision of a physician and issue prescriptions on their own. Alarm has already been expressed that such centers are contributing to the inappropriate prescription of antibiotics for upper respiratory tract conditions, which in some locations accounted for 54% of all patient visits.[48] To avoid potential adverse legal liability, the centers most often post-visit offer referral of the patient to their network emergency room at the hospital for follow-up care, but the outcome for many may not accomplish this goal (see vignette below). These concerns and similar problems will tend to grow if physicians continue to be replaced in this health care setting. Whereas the author may see the logic of the urgent care center approach for the young patient with minimal comorbidities that do not demand a comprehensive in-depth view of the patient, he is somewhat skeptical of elderly patients receiving a clear analysis of their problems within the context of the comorbidity limitations they carry and the impact of the problem being examined. The elderly may be at higher risk of unappreciated complications (e.g., drug interactions, missed diagnoses, Clostridium difficile overgrowth, etc.) in being evaluated in such a system if not seen by a more experienced health care provider. These aspects will have to be borne in mind by the elderly patient accessing such health care providers. Future studies and follow up will undoubtedly clarify the risk/benefit of such an approach to the elderly patient.

Vignette Case
—————————— ⸙ ——————————

An 88-year-old man well known in the author's city as a prominent businessman to many, joined his peer group every Monday evening in the city's most well-known men's club for dinner to share stories and past experiences. Unfortunately, he suffered the comorbidity of COPD and was utilizing supplemental oxygen cannisters for ambulatory movement. His history of smoking Pall Mall cigarettes during his youth was known to many. History of details obtained from his companion, revealed that to avoid some personal embarrassment, he went to the men's bathroom without his oxygen cannister, and was found by two of his peers on the bathroom floor confused. They called for an ambulance and cleaned blood from around his mouth and an abrasion on his forehead. The ambulance arrived, emergency medical technicians followed the procedures of the city, and they transported him to the nearest medical site, which was an urgent care center of one of the largest hospital health care systems. Subsequently, after evaluation, he was sent home without any explicit instructions and received written directions to see his physician or return to the ACO hospital emergency room if problems developed. Two weeks later he was found to have died during the night, the cause of death was established as a cerebral subdural hematoma. The visit to the urgent care center had failed to appreciate that this elderly man undoubtedly had atherosclerotic disease with his COPD, and that falls in this elderly group can allow a small artery bleed to be held open by stiff vessels within the brain. The slow leakage of blood built up a clot between the skull and brain tissue, that slowly collapsed a chamber within the brain leading to death. The recognition of his comorbidities was not appreciated or went unnoticed, a brain MRI or CT was not obtained relatively soon, and subsequently an error in judgment led to an early death.

Many explanations could account for this chain of events. Was the patient seen by an allied health person or a physician? Was the physician relatively young or older with experience? Was the patient given instructions to follow up at the hospital for a CT or MRI? Did the family or companion not recognize the seriousness of the situation from a lack of health knowledge of the patient's risk?

This case illustrates that in 2020 urgent care centers can pose potential dangers to the elderly. While suturing a peripheral laceration or treating an abrasion may be perfectly adequate without consequences, the comorbidities of the elderly demand careful consideration and physical examination at every health encounter. It cannot be a matter of brief efficient beneficial pass-through for patient or family convenience without weighing the risks of the patient in the context of their existing health status, frailty, or comorbidities.

Lastly, is the entrance of health insurers (Aetna) that have been acquired by large pharmaceutical chains (CVS Health Corporation) to offering free "Minute Clinic" visits without co-pay available at the drugstore's chain pharmacies. Other developments initiated by health insurers include offering their own primary care centers to ensure patients are retained within their health care system to guide referrals and save costs. How these models will ultimately affect the elderly is unclear, but they are currently ongoing. These methods of health care delivery are being organized to retain patients within a certain health care system and provide cost savings to the patient and the health care system. The elderly would be well advised to know their own comorbidities and risk factors prior to such visits, provide their history and discuss it openly when being evaluated during such encounters.

PART II.

THE ELDERLY HEALTH PYRAMID

CHAPTER SIX

Introduction to Part II

Precision Medicine

IN THE CURRENT era with the innovations in genetics and technologies, many physicians aspire to attain precision clinical medicine in individual patients. The goal is to treat each patient as an individual with distinct genetic, biological, and social determinant factors that affect susceptibility to disease, treatment responses, and adherence to therapies.[49] This **precision medicine** utilizes huge amounts of individual and population data to discover and deliver the right treatment to the right patient at the right time. As a result, large national studies such as the National Institutes of Health Precision Medicine Initiative and the United Kingdom Biobank have been formed with precision medicine as a major goal.[49] One early NIH initiative in this arena is precision nutrition.[50] It is a multifaceted interventional approach that goes beyond choosing healthy foods. Poor nutrition is a key risk factor for a host of chronic diseases and conditions that are the leading causes of death and disability in the US—including cardiovascular disease and stroke, type 2 diabetes, obesity, cancers, and others—with associated health care costs estimated in the hundreds of billions of dollars annually.[51] The role of this initiative is to spur research to define the role of nutrition in promoting health and reducing the burden of disease throughout life and across generations. This research is especially important in view of the current COVID-19 pandemic exposure of the increased risks faced by people with underlying conditions who have been disproportionately affected as a vulnerable population due to health and social disparities. One must wonder how poor or incorrect nutrition is affecting our inherent immune system during the pandemic, particularly when we have recent knowledge of the dietary inflammatory potential of non-plant based diets.[50]

Similarly, it is also apparent that this approach has given impetus to the emerging field of wearable health care technologies in the form of data gathering watches or smartphone devices to provide individualized data for identifying exercise and sleep patterns, diet variations, environmental changes, and trends of health variance and/or early maladies.[52] These emerging precision developments in the health sciences are in their infancy. Nevertheless, early targeting to identify changes in SpO2 (for sleep apnea and COVID-19 respiratory decline), heart rate and rhythm (for atrial fibrillation), body positional accelerometer (to detect falls, exercise and sleep patterns) and glucose levels (diabetes management) currently exist.[52, 53] But as shown in one of the earliest population studies (Apple watch 419,000 persons), improved study design to identify the appropriate populations who gain the greatest benefit will be needed in the marketplace to help define their promising value.[54]

Social Determinants of Health

Whereas, definite information is required by each elderly patient to set his individual preventive and/or surveillance health program to deal with his current state of health and recognized comorbidities (or wellness), certain elements in each elder's life are vitally important. These elements consist not only of preventive and clinical medicine, but also of personal fiscal security and a safe environment that affords community and/or other companionship (Figure 8). Attention during the last decade has been drawn to these **social determinants of health** which describe the social, environmental, and economic circumstances

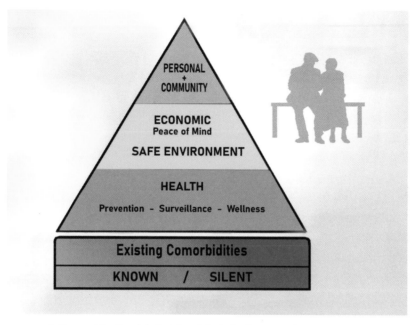

FIGURE 8. Pyramid of health for the elderly built upon their existing comorbidities.

in which people live and work, thereby influencing their health and quality of life[55, 56] "Poly-social risk scores" from large datasets that capture the interaction of multiple social determinants with the ongoing investigations of the complex diverse genetic base (existing in the US) of each individual are now garnering scientific attention.[57] In some circumstances the social determinants explain more of the variance in health care outcomes and disparities than the traditional access to or quality of the medical care.[55] The final chapters of this primer will examine some of these social determinant components of health and lifestyle, economic peace of mind and safety, and community and companionship to present some aspects that seem unique to the elderly in America. They will point out medical, government, and social services that are available to aid them in their personal program.

Ageism

Ageism is defined as a stereotyping of, prejudice or discrimination against a particular age-group, especially the elderly. The first known usage of this term was in 1969, and since 2016, it has been recognized as a risk factor to individual health by the World Health Organization.[58] Ageism is highly prevalent, socially accepted, and usually unchallenged because of its largely implicit and subconscious nature.[58]

Over the years, this attitude has emerged from several perspectives within our society. For example, Graham Sutherland, the famous English portrait painter whose unflattering painting of Winston Churchill drew the subject's ire, is supposed to have remarked to Churchill that "Age is cruel!" Reality and expectation of aging is one's individual perspective, but the author would argue that in 2020, ageism is a devaluation of both the aged elder as well as the aging life cycle. As we become older we experience ageism not only from others, but also from ourselves.

Popular women's magazines such as *Cosmopolitan*, *Vogue*, and *Harper's Bazaar* began in the 1970s to encourage women to resist the process of aging by seeking a more youthful (and sexual) appearance. Their marketing and advertising strategies promoted an empire of beauty products, the expansion of plastic surgery into cosmetic surgery, and by the end of the twentieth century an array of nail/hair salons and day spas across the US. Celebrities of the day in the entertainment industry also devalued aging at a time when the women's liberation movement focused increasingly on the emerging career woman. These factors, directed particularly at women, slowly devalued the aging process during one's life cycle and dulled the value of an aged appearance and the wisdom that comes with aging. To some US women the fear of a "younger woman" eager to become a "trophy wife" threatened their spousal bliss, and became the rationale for adopting this new standard of beauty, health, and happiness.

These attitudinal changes were also foisted upon men by commercial products and procedures, as well as the processes described above. Pharmaceutical products like Rogaine or hair implantations promised to preserve hair; the use of sildenafil (Viagra) and supplemental testosterone extended virility; and vitamin/protein supplements were alleged to help men to appear younger. Some men, like women, opted for cosmetic surgery to improve their appearance. By the end of the twentieth century, these superficial efforts to defy aging were also expressed in the economic life cycle of individual men with the onset of the digital century. The economic recession of 2008 displaced many men in their late fifties 50s and 60s from their jobs, particularly those associated with the business structures of the twentieth century (i.e., personal secretaries, managerial positions, etc.). Many found it difficult to compete in the new digital century with younger recruits who came armed with digital skills and entrepreneurial energy inspired by emerging icons of millennial billionaires (Mark Zuckerberg, Jeff Bezos, and Elon Musk). Many realized their job skills were devalued in the digital era, and all too often they had to accept a decline in their overall value in the job market. This acceptance of lower paying positions by large numbers of middle-aged men contributed to the devaluation of the middle class.[59, 60] Unfortunately, experiencing this cascade of change led to depression in some, rather than taking pride in the accomplishment of aging in a competitive society.

Vignette

—————————— ❧ ——————————

A University of Michigan National Poll of Health Aging examined older adults' experiences with nine forms of everyday ageism. These forms were categorized into three groups: (1) exposure to ageist messages, (2) ageism in interpersonal interactions, and (3) internalized ageism (personally held beliefs about aging and older people).

"Overall, 82% of older adults reported regularly experiencing at least one form of everyday ageism in their day-to-day lives.[61] Two in three older adults (65%) reported exposure to ageist messages in their day-to-day lives. This included often or sometimes hearing, seeing, and/or reading jokes about old age, aging, or older people (61%) or hearing, seeing, and/or reading things suggesting that older adults and aging are unattractive or undesirable (38%)."[61]

"Nearly half of older adults (45%) reported experiencing ageism in their interpersonal interactions. Specific experiences included other people often or sometimes assuming that because of their age, they have difficulty using cell phones and computers (22%), hearing and/or seeing (17%), or remembering and/or understanding (17%). Some older adults also reported that others assume they do not do anything important or valuable (15%) or that they need help with tasks they can do on their own (15%)."[61]

Unfortunately, until the onset of the pandemic of COVID-19, the World Health Organization, while acknowledging ageism as a socially unacceptable form of discrimination and prejudice, had not previously focused much attention on it. With COVID-19, it became obvious that ageism was a major factor impacting health care delivery and outcomes in the initial phases of the pandemic. In the early phase of COVID-19, researchers realized that 80% of US deaths had occurred in those over 65 years of age, but later they came to appreciate that neither co-morbidities nor the social determinants of disease were the only factors affecting the elderly.[59] Whereas early jokes in the media referred to the pandemic as a hashtag, #BoomerRemover, some state officials suggested that those over 70 years of age "sacrifice" themselves for the good of the economy.[62] Early statistics revealed that more than one-third to 40% of total US deaths occurred in the 1.5 million residents living in one of the approximately 15,600 US nursing or long-term care facilities.[59, 62]

These attitudes toward older Americans reflected the general devaluing of the elderly in the late twentieth and early twenty-first centuries. This devaluation of older lives led to discussions of triaging in times of medical shortages and emerged in the discourse of medical care decisions during COVID-19 in some US states.[62] This factor unfortunately may be particularly germane to men who seem more susceptible to COVID-19, experience greater severity of disease, and do not fare well with frailty when the disease is prolonged as compared to women.

Hopefully, the concepts discussed above contribute to a fuller understanding of one's personal individual health status, co-morbidities, varying work/environmental circumstances, and individual risks of social determinants of health and ageism. They offer a framework for planning and practicing a personal health program going forward. The elderly should be alert to the seeming devaluation of their importance in some aspects of today's COVID-19 society. It is another form of "unintentional injury" to their individual health that has emerged during the pandemic that must be guarded against when possible.

Shared Decision Making

Most elders in the US can reflect back over the past thirty to forty years on specific interactions they have had with the health care system, most of which required a one-on-one discussion with their personal physician.

These discussions were usually brief without decision sharing but offered an explanation of the physician's opinion and a course of action. Then came the appearance of operative permits for surgical procedures, and then patients were required to sign procedural permits for specific diagnostic procedures (e.g. cardiac catheterizations, colonoscopies, endoscopy, etc.). Subsequently, hospitals required patients to confirm the existence of a living will before admitting them for care. Physicians required patients to take more responsibility for their medical decisions out of concern for potential litigation over or liability for risks associated with such diagnostic or therapeutic procedures or hospitalization. At this point, it was incumbent on the physician to explain the risk and benefit of the diagnostic test or the medical procedure, but there usually was limited participation by the patient in the decision making. It was a yes or no decision. With limited health literacy in the last century, most often these decisions were rendered by the physician.

In the past, most Americans agreed that "the doctor knows best." The author believes that adage is outdated and does not apply to the elder of today. With the increasing complexity of medical diagnostic tests, medical treatments, the associated medical costs, and the advancing medical knowledge of patients, the patients' decisions and interactions about many facets of their health care matters. This aspect of health care is just evolving in the twenty-first century; weighing the risk/benefit ratio of any specific diagnostic test or treatment course is an important aspect of the doctor-patient relationship. The knowledge of the risks of a diagnostic procedure, the possible benefit gained by that procedure, and the patient's fears or anxieties associated with the procedure must be shared by both the physician and the patient.[63, 64]

Shared decision making has been advancing within mainstream cardiovascular medicine for many years concerning implantable devices (e.g. pacemakers and implantable cardioverter defibrillators) and medications. Anticoagulation and the use of medical devices are particularly germane to the elderly who fear change of body image or increased bleeding hazards. A physician should present these matters to patients, when cognition and life expectancy of the patient are appropriate, so that the patient's values and preference in health care are part of the decision. Physicians should seek to align medical care choices and goals with each patient's personal decision and care. The author feels fortified in this process by practicing evidence-based medicine guided on outcome data where it exists and sharing uncertainty with the patient when such data does not exist. Judgment must be exercised by both the physician and the patient; such collaboration defines the physician-patient relationship. The elder must gain education and literacy about their own health to ensure continuing decision-making capability, a good quality of life, and the ability to render sound judgment.

CHAPTER SEVEN

Prevention, Surveillance, and Wellness

Prevention

PREVENTION IN THE medical sense embraces the concept of
(1) **primary prevention**, that is prevention of the onset of a disease, involving interventions that are applied before there is any
evidence of disease or injury; (2) **secondary prevention**, measures are meant to stabilize, regress, and mitigate an ongoing
existing disease process; and (3) **tertiary prevention**, which is
aimed at reducing the negative impact of an established disease
by restoring function and reducing disease-related complications. Medical progress of both science and methods change
over time, and that, unfortunately, may lead to confusion in
the population at large. A good example is the case of aspirin
introduced as early as the 1950s to render benefit against heart
attacks and stroke. Physicians came to realize that aspirins'
antithrombotic action was beneficial in the spontaneous erosion or rupture of an atherosclerotic plaque involved in the
process of heart attacks and stroke. But with the aging of the
population and the increased number of elderly patients, the
adverse risks of bleeding and limited benefit in those over 75
years became apparent.[65, 66] This controversy, which surfaced
in the last two years, is still incompletely defined despite recommendations from the American College of Cardiology and
the American Heart Association.[67] Not to be overlooked is the
prevention of colorectal cancer in those families with a history

of the disease. The lifetime benefit of reducing colon cancer in a dose-dependent manner is a side benefit of aspirin in addition to its cardiovascular benefits.[68] A recent investigation by meta-analysis of more than 130,000 individuals (from 13 randomized clinical trials) has shown that the associated risk of intracranial hemorrhage with low-dose aspirin is confined to those of Asian race or ethnicity or low body mass index (BMI).[69] Therefore, the decision to take low-dose aspirin should be decided by the patient and physician, weighing the individual risk/benefit for the individual elder taking into account multiple factors.

Similarly, fewer than 2% of 186,854 participants in 28 statin trials were older than 75 years, and suspicion of the non-benefit of statins arose as to the primary prevention benefit in an elderly population. Recent evidence from 327,000 eligible US veterans 75 years and older who were initially started on new statin usage showed a 25% reduction in all-cause mortality and 20% reduction in cardiovascular mortality.[70]

Notwithstanding these **primary prevention** recommendations, aspirin and statins are also **secondary preventive** agents. If a patient has evidence of an atherosclerotic process (e.g., past heart attack, stroke, peripheral artery disease, etc.) aspirin is often prescribed to limit ongoing disease and is indicated.[67] Several pharmaceuticals serve as both primary and secondary preventive agents. They include many statins, blood pressure lowering agents, and agents treating metabolic syndromes. A recent **tertiary preventive** agent that is widely promoted in a television ad is Entresto (sacubitril/valsartan), which is recommended only in stabilized heart failure patients to reduce new events (negative impact). As recently described, despite the presence of twelve new secondary preventive agents in 2020, 80% of patients with ischemic heart disease, and 99% of those with prior heart attack (myocardial infarction) were eligible to receive at least one new preventive drug.[71] However, the scientific breakthroughs of the last decade remain largely unrealized for most eligible patients because of poor appreciation by the medical community, lack of health knowledge in the general population, prohibitive costs (ranging from \$14,000 to \$200,000/year), and difficult authorization policies and/or high patient copays within health care systems.[71] Many medical therapies, however, are very affordable, cost-effective, and within the budget of the elderly. Moreover, the pharmaceutical industry has created compassionate use programs to assist in the cost of some medications for patients in need. Nevertheless, because of comorbidities that occur throughout life in becoming elderly, one must anticipate that their own individual medical regimen may require both primary and secondary pharmaceuticals and preventive lifestyle choices to preserve a healthy state of being well or achieving wellness.

Surveillance

SURVEILLANCE means "close watch kept over someone or something (as by a detective)." That is exactly what each of us would love to have regarding our health most of our lives. In the *formative* years, parents provide this surveillance of a child's health, and the author has found that today parental surveillance often extends into the child's young adulthood. Indeed, the ACA allows young adults to be covered under their parents' insurance plan to age 26 years. However, since the establishment of Medicare, preventive and medical surveillance for older people has become disjointed and is constantly undergoing change. As discussed earlier, the Framingham project introduced the concept of tracking medical history and examinations (physical and blood) to follow a population.[23] It soon became clear to the medical field that primary prevention or secondary prevention demanded a minimum of a history and physical examination accompanied by blood studies. From the 1960s to the 1980s, many health diagnostic assessments required only an ECG (electrocardiogram) and chest x-ray. Whether for an individual diagnostic reason or an insurance exam, this kind of assessment was not viewed as a preventive modality or provided for by insurance or government services. The US Preventive Task Force was initiated in 1984, and its guidelines eventually evolved into policies adopted by Congress. The Task Force, an independent advisory panel that conducts impartial assessments of scientific evidence, submits its recommendations to Congress annually.[72] Although sponsored by the government, the Task Force does not represent a specific organization or US government agency. Its views are independent. The Medicare, Medicaid, and SCHIP Benefits Improvement and Protection Act of 2000 authorized the government to pay for preventive health care services. These benefits are easily accessible online. (https://www.healthcare.gov/coverage/preventive-care-benefits/).

This act marked the beginning of preventive surveillance in the US. Every elder today is provided by Medicare a cost-free annual wellness examination with blood studies as indicated by the physician. At this examination, the physician should review the elder's status and offer guidance on vaccines and medications. Based on the author's experience, these available cost-free services are markedly underutilized by the current elderly population.

Simultaneously, new technological discoveries within the field of medicine have made possible increased medical surveillance for an established disease process. Innovations include medical imaging with ultrasound (echo) studies, radioisotope scans, computerized tomographic (CT) scans, and the magnetic resonance imaging (MRI) examination. These technologies in the twenty-first century provide insights that were in their infancy in the last century, and physicians quickly realized that monitoring an aggressive disease process was firmly aided by not only blood studies, but also by following progressive functional and anatomical modalities of the disease. Today these medical surveillance strategies are being utilized to detect a serious disease at an early stage to limit disability and early death in some specific sub-populations exhibiting high-risk factors. This is the case for lung cancer screening for adults 50 to 80 years at high risk of lung cancer because they were heavy smokers or have quit in the past fifteen years.[73] Medicare provides this examination as one of its benefits (https://www.healthcare.gov/coverage/preventive-care-benefits/). Despite the availability of Medicare or other insurance coverage, the elderly patient must adopt a lifestyle of periodic surveillance consistent with their individual risks and known comorbidities. Along the actuarial curve of aging, the incidence of increasing risk of disease with aging is real, and although we do not live forever, sustaining the prevention of disability and maintaining the quality of life are our goals.

Wellness

WELLNESS is difficult to define, especially for the elderly. The dictionary states that it is "the quality or state of being in good health especially as an active sought goal." The elderly often hear from their peers, "you look so well." But outward appearances can be deceptive. The exterior well-looking body can portray itself as functioning and appearing "well," but it may be suffering low back pain every morning, loss of bladder control, insomnia, or some other chronic malady. As discussed above in the social determinants of disease (Figure 8 on page 45), the anxiety of living within an unsafe environment of gun violence, suffering the loneliness of no social contact, poor individual shelter, or lack of good nutrition due to lack of fiscal resources, all take a toll on our state of wellness. Happiness in life for many elders is found to be messy; personal contentment with peace of mind would be bliss for most of the elderly.

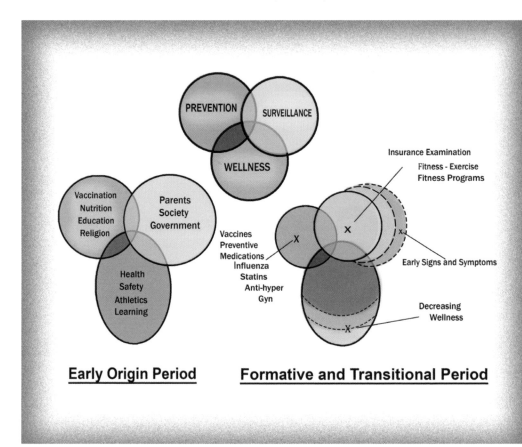

FIGURE 9A. Prevention, surveillance, and wellness – *early origin* period and *formative-transitional* period.

The goal of this primer is to offer a minimum prescription for readers in the US to follow to define their personal risk factors, comorbidities, and gain the preventive and medical knowledge to achieve wellness. As shown in Figure 9a and 9b (above), the balance of prevention, surveillance, and wellness must be individually set by each elder to attain that pyramid of optimal health. The American Heart Association and the Cancer Society have clearly indicated the greatest causes of mortality

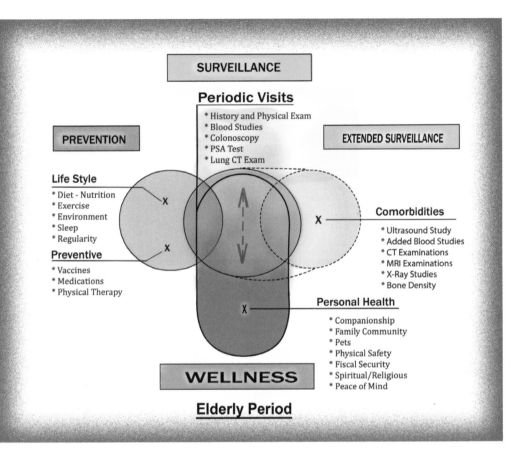

FIGURE 9B. Prevention, surveillance, and wellness in the elderly. Important ongoing factors during the *elderly* life cycle period.

and morbidity currently existing in the US are diseases of the heart and malignant neoplasms or cancer. As noted in Table 2, accidents (unintentional injuries e.g., elderly falls), chronic lower respiratory diseases (COPD and emphysema), and cerebrovascular diseases (strokes) round out the most prevalent imminent threats to the elderly.[74] Specific recommendations in this regard are addressed for both men and women in the following sections of the primer.

TABLE 2. Leading causes of death in the United States.

Leading Causes of Death in the United States

1.	Diseases of heart (heart disease)
2.	Malignant neoplasms (cancer)
3.	Accidents (unintentional injuries)
4.	Chronic lower respiratory diseases (COPD and emphysema)
5.	Cerebrovascular diseases (strokes)
6.	Alzheimer disease
7.	Diabetes mellitus
8.	Influenza and pneumonia
9.	Kidney disease
10.	Intentional self-harm (suicide)

Adapted from Kochanek KD et al.[74]

CHAPTER EIGHT

Genetics, Lifestyle, and Preventive Measures

Genetics

AS CAN BE gathered from Part I, each individual elder should know the diseases of his parents and grandparents if possible. They define his genetic risks. Particularly in America this is the starting point of every physician's assessment to gauge the potential problems of a patient. The leading causes of death in the US include heart disease and stroke, hypertension, cancer, and diabetes, but knowing the patient's family history places the patient's risk in context and indicates what they should be examined for in the beginning. Genetic predisposition constitutes approximately 30% of the risk for an early death but can be modified by individual lifestyle choices and behavior.[6,75] This history-taking introduces the elder to the existence of his possible "risk factors" which may be detected or disclosed during his examination. For example, the presence of heart disease and stroke, hypertension and diabetes indicate the process of atherosclerosis which affects all the vasculature of the body and can affect the development of kidney disease or peripheral artery disease as well. A family history of prostate or colon cancer or aneurysm is also very predictive of an individual's hereditary risk of those abnormalities occurring. Common genetic diseases which can be inherited and influence an individual's risk as a man is listed in Table 3 on page 62 and as a woman in Table 5 on page 104. Other risk factors are acquired through life in the adoption of an individual's lifestyle and preventive practices.

TABLE 3. Risk factors for elderly men.

Genetic risk factors	Acquired risk factors
Atherosclerosis – heart attack (coronary artery disease), stroke (cerebrovascular disease). and peripheral artery disease	Tobacco usage – cigarette smoking, chewing tobacco
Hypertension – high blood pressure	Sedentary lifestyle – lack of exercise and activity
Hyperlipidemia – elevated cholesterol or triglycerides	Frailty – unintentional weight loss, exhaustion, weakness (grip strength), slow walking speed, and low physical activity.
Colon cancer – colon or rectal polyps	Obesity
Prostate cancer – elevated PSA	Against vaccines and/or preventive medications
Diabetes mellitus – elevated glucose or HbA1C	Alcoholism
Obesity	Substance abuse

Genetics impart a major physiological and physical variable which indirectly influences the pattern and rate of aging. This occurs even within first degree family members when a physician encounters a petite daughter with thin characteristics and a robust son with stocky characteristics. In the 1940s, William Sheldon, a psychologist, used body types to help classify personalities.[76] Ectomorphic, characterized as thin, weak, and usually tall, he described as intelligent, gentle, and calm, but self-conscious,

TABLE 4. Key guidelines of exercise for older adults.

The key guidelines for adults also apply to older adults. In addition the following key guidelines are just for older adults:

As part of their weekly physical activity, older adults should do multicomponent physical activity that includes balance training as well as aerobic and muscle-strengthening activities.

Older adults should determine their level of effort for physical activity relative to their level of fitness.

When older adults cannot do 150 minutes of moderate-intensity aerobic activity a week because of chronic conditions, they should be as physically active as their abilities and conditions allow.

KEY GUIDELINES OF EXERCISE FOR ADULTS

Adults should move more and sit less throughout the day. Some physical activity is better than none. Adults who sit less and do any amount of moderate-to-vigorous physical activity gain some health benefits.

For substantial health benefits, adults should do at least 150 minutes (2 hours and 30 minutes) to 300 minutes (5 hours) a week of moderate-intensity, or 75 minutes (1 hour and 15 minutes) to 150 minutes (2 hours and 30 minutes) a week of vigorous-intensity aerobic physical activity, or an equivalent combination of moderate and vigorous-intensity aerobic activity.

Preferably, aerobic activity should be spread throughout the week.

Additional health benefits are gained by doing physical activity beyond the equivalent of 300 minutes (5 hours) of moderate-intensity physical activity a week.

Adults should also do muscle-strengthening activities of moderate or greater intensity that involve all major muscle groups on 2 or more days a week, as these activities provide additional health benefits.

Adapted from Piercy KL, et al. [90]

introverted, and anxious. Mesomorphic, characterized as hard, muscular, thick-skinned, and as having good posture, he described as competitive, extroverted, and tough. And Endomorphic, characterized as fat, usually short, and having difficulty losing weight, he described as outgoing, friendly, happy, and laid-back, but also lazy and selfish.[76] This physiological variability within the same family accounts for different health profiles, as the author's experience with the two siblings suggests. The daughter at age 72 years is active and appears younger than her stated age, while the son at age 65 years has developed a protruding abdomen with fat and has developed diabetes (adult type) that was not previously known to be within the family. This genetic physiological variation manifested within a family by genetics results in markedly different risks of future disease.

The author has always been most mindful of the patient's sex and inheritable factors in trying to determine their biological age versus their chronological age.[77] After all, women have always enjoyed a higher life expectancy than men. Since cardiovascular disease is the major determinant of death in the US, both the sex of the patient and the family history give clues to their vascular aging. Data show that family history of cardiovascular disease increases the risk from 40% to 75% dependent on the degree of relatedness.[78] When one focuses only on cardiovascular disease and its vascular components, the complex interplay of one's heredity and chronological aging interacting with all of the other aspects described in this primer is apparent.[77]

Lifestyle

It has been said anonymously that "wealth is the number of days that an individual can live in the lifestyle he is accustomed to." Of course, Americans strive in a capitalistic society to have a lifestyle somewhat above what they were accustomed to. Compared to Europeans, Americans focus on work and have more constricted vacations and more restricted travel. Their lives in some ways have been put on hold until they retire.[4] As shown in Figure 9 in the previous chapter, their wellness may have decreased in the *formative* and *transitional* periods of life, and now as elderly persons they may require ongoing extended surveillance and medical therapies for comorbidities (known or unknown). This will and can affect their lifestyle. As stated earlier, medical advances have attached an additional thirty years onto their elderly period; in short, "old age got longer."[4]

Having this perspective in mind, the most basic factors in lifestyle to examine, modify if necessary, and address as an elder include diet, exercise, environment, and sleep. The elderly must become aware through the regularity of their lifestyle of their own personal physical and mental resilience, a measure, if you will, of personal reserve.

Diet and nutrition

Unequivocally at this time in the life cycle, the author advises an elder to follow the Mediterranean diet, because of its proven benefit.[79] It not only is associated with the prevention of heart disease, but also reduced mortality for all cardiovascular disease (including stroke) and cancer as well. Although an elderly person's diet is shaped by a life-long set of preferences, adopting a Mediterranean diet from the age of 65 years could help the individual to avoid late life cognitive impairment and frailty.[80, 81, 82] Associated benefit on risk factors by the Mediterranean diet is thought to extend the period of health while you are aging. A major constituent of the diet receiving attention is olive oil, which helps in preventing negative cardiovascular outcomes.[83] As others have pointed out, the diet does not exist in a vacuum; it evolved culturally as a way of life in which cooking was central to family, friendship, and a sense of community.[82] For more than three decades, the data show that these benefits are unequivocal, and the Mediterranean diet can easily be varied to afford weight loss.[79] Although recent data have shown that a low-fat vegan diet leads to greater weight loss (by 6.4 Kg) compared to a Mediterranean diet, with no difference in blood lipids, it was found that both systolic and diastolic blood pressure decreased more on the Mediterranean diet (by 6.0 and 3.2 mmHg, respectively).[84] Considering the fact that treating hypertension (high blood pressure) is the number one goal of the Global Burden of Disease, the Mediterranean diet would seem to be the ongoing "best choice" for most US elderly.[26, 27, 28]

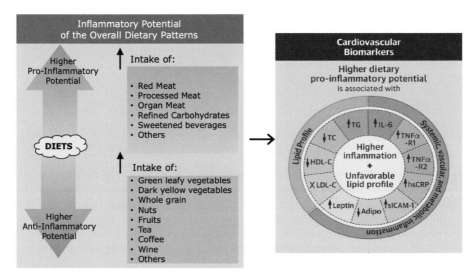

FIGURE 10. Diets and their inflammatory effects on cardiovascular biomarkers of risk. Adapted from Li J, et al.[87]

Elders, knowing that loss of muscle mass occurs with aging in their late 70s and early 80s, should give more attention to increasing sources of protein in the Mediterranean diet. Almonds, walnuts, and nuts in general have been regarded as sources of beneficial protein affecting decreased deaths due to cancer, heart disease, and respiratory disease.[85, 86] Medical researchers in more recent times have established the benefit of all plant-based diets, as they have anti-inflammatory properties and decrease inflammatory biomarkers, which is a critical mechanism against atherothrombosis. Sustained walnut ingestion (over 2 years) has also been shown in randomized trials to lower adverse lipid patterns and reduce cardiovascular disease outcomes (Figure 10).[87, 88]

In the medical era of the last century, eggs were portrayed as a villainous source of cholesterol. Now in the twenty-first century, eggs can be a good source of protein for elders, many of whom are on statins anyway. Older people should limit themselves to one egg a day, which should have no adverse effects on blood lipids, cardiovascular disease, or mortality.[89] The author has recommended eggs to those patients who have noted their individual loss of muscle mass and are seeking sources of quality protein.

Finally, alcoholic intake and its effects must also be addressed. Moderation has been the medical advice over the course of your life, but between 65 and 90 years individuals will experience different phenomena depending on the comorbidities they have brought to the age. With aging, the direct effect of previous intake and tolerance will be affected by decreasing muscle mass and possible liver dysfunction. The twenty-four hours after imbibing alcohol will be accompanied by decreased sport performance (i.e., less weightlifting strength, earlier running fatigue, etc.) and a certain listlessness. By age 75 years these changes are apparent to most elders. If they brought the comorbidity of susceptibility to atrial fibrillation, it is in danger of being provoked by alcohol. Elders must learn individually their new alcohol tolerance. The presence of liver abnormality (e.g., fatty liver) can make these observations occur even earlier (age 50 to 60 years). Not only does the liver decrease its ability to metabolize the alcohol (resulting in the listlessness or fatigue lasting longer), but the decreased muscle mass, which also metabolizes alcohol, cannot process it quickly. If you suffer the comorbidity of heart failure, that could also be made worse in the succeeding twenty-four hours after imbibing alcohol.

Multiple processes are in play; therefore, prudence suggests that the elder must decrease individual alcoholic intake with aging and comorbidities, acknowledge its persisting effect into the following day, and plan accordingly for the intake of alcohol.

Exercise

All elders need exercise, regardless of their age, to insure functionality, wellness, and personal reserve. **Personal reserve** as defined by the author is the body's ability to isolate a disease process or injury, address its treatment, and recover one's state of wellness. *It embodies an aspect of physical fitness, baseline good health, and reserve immunity.* Aspects of regular physical activity have health benefits for everyone. Some benefits occur immediately, such as reduced feelings of anxiety, reduced blood pressure, and improved sleep, cognitive function, and insulin sensitivity. Other benefits, such as increased cardiorespiratory fitness, increased muscle strength, decreased depression symptoms, and sustained reduction in blood pressure accrue over months or years of physical activity.[90] At all levels of blood pressure (including those with hypertension), the risk of cardiovascular events is significantly reduced whatever the level of physical activity achieved.[91] At the elder level the physical activity must be embedded in their lifestyle, ready to encounter a threat to wellness. Exercise for the elder must be gauged for safety within the limits of their comorbidities. Realizing that the current generation of elders has had an escalating number of hip and knee replacements from the "marathon" and "iron man" competitions of the baby boomer generation, avoidance of falls (third leading cause of deaths as unintentional injuries), should be a key ingredient to individual programs. The author supports an embedded program of Tai Chi or selected Pilates exercises complementing multicomponent physical activity as called for in the Physical Activity Guidelines for Americans of the US Office of Disease Prevention and Health Promotion.[90, 92] These recommendations for all adults and the elderly are shown in Table 4 on page 63. Notwithstanding the limitations of the American landscape with the need for travel by vehicle (instead of village or neighborhood walking such as in Europe), the guidelines provided indicate dynamic walking as its main recommendation. Recognizing the difference between European and American ways of life, the guidelines encourage walking in covered shopping centers and school track venues, which are common in the US. Recent studies have drawn attention to the increased number of hours individuals spend sitting, due to technologies that encourage sedentary behavior; such habits have been associated with increased morbidities and mortality, and undoubtedly account for the multiple digital fitness apps which urge one to stand hourly.[93] The National Institute on Aging NIH site presents useful guidelines concerning exercise at: https://www.nia.nih.gov/health/exercise-physical-activity.

The author has found this approach generally applicable until people are in their 80s, when many have lost vertebral height (loss of vertebral disc cartilage with low back pain or vertebral osteoporosis), experienced a restricted gait (smaller step secondary to hip fibrosis, replacement, or disease), and are susceptible to balance problems (from visual or hearing problems, and loss of feeling {proprioception} in feet with weaker leg strength (Figure 11). These aging features now so common in today's elders have led to falls becoming a leading cause of death in the elderly.[94] This is the time of onset of frailty (discussed below). Twenty-nine percent of elders fall once a year, and 10% fall twice annually.[94] Twenty to 30% of those who fall sustain moderate to severe injury, resulting in more than 30,000 deaths and 800,000 hospitalizations annually.[95] Deficits in gait and balance are the most prominent risk factors, but some medications may

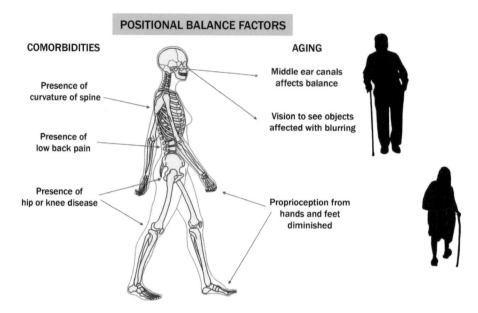

FIGURE 11. Positional balance factors associated with falls. Adapted from Motifolio, Inc.

also contribute to this outcome. Early study of multifactorial interventions (STRIDE trial), administered by nurses, unfortunately shows they have not significantly lowered the rate of a serious fall injury in a primary care setting.[95] In this age group with these comorbidities looming, the author advises "medical" Tai Chi to establish strength and balance while slowly improving osteoarthritic and fibrotic joints and vertebrae.[96] These exercises can be performed in twenty minutes and are easily performed two to three times a week. Tai Chi can be coupled with a multicomponent physical activity plan that is individualized to avoid inactivity. Inactivity has been shown in population studies to be directly deleterious in the form of creating increased heart disease and stroke (Figure 12).[97]

One final caveat is for those men who came under the influence of the "macho" era of baby boomer ironman competitions, Rambo movies, and other extreme training that

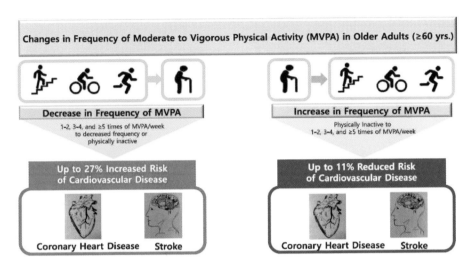

FIGURE 12. Changes in exercise frequency and cardiovascular outcomes in older adults. Adapted from Kim K, et al.[97]

tended to push individuals to the maximum physical exertion in whatever exercises were chosen. Recent data of more than 400,000 *transitional* individuals followed for seven years into their 60s have shown stark differences between men and women.[98] Whereas women can benefit greatly from such maximal exercises, especially in avoiding cardiac arrhythmias such as atrial fibrillation, men at high levels are subject to an increase in factors leading to more complications including atrial fibrillation (Figure 13).[98, 99]

Nevertheless, recent data from the National Health Interview Survey of 403,681 participants who provided data on self-reported physical activity showed that vigorous activity lowered all-cause mortality by 17% as compared to the same total measurement of moderate activity. There were similar outcomes for cardiovascular and cancer mortality.[100] Clinicians and public health educators were urged to recommend 150 minutes or more per week of either moderate or vigorous physical activity to maximize population health and wellness.[100]

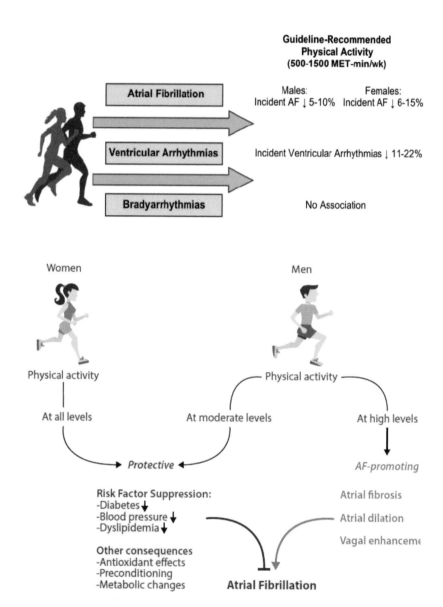

FIGURE 13. Associations between physical activity and development of cardiac arrhythmias. Adapted from Elliott AD, et al.[98] and Nattel S.[99]

Environment

The environment affects all prevention and is crucial in achieving positive health outcomes in the elderly. Consider the so called perfect "blue zones" of old age. One such area is the island of Ikaria in Greece. This island provides fresh vegetables and a locally produced food supply, clean unpolluted air, a non-hostile environment free from violence or threat from crime, no workplace stress, blissful quiet, supportive community, and beautiful natural surroundings. It provides the individual an opportunity to establish one's own regularity (see below). Of course, life does not provide such havens to most of us. But many Americans seek idealized settings across the country to provide components of a healthful retirement or place of living, especially as they age. The social determinants of disease (e.g., being close to children or grandchildren, need to work, etc.) all influence the environment elders choose. This subject will be discussed more extensively later in the section on personal wellness.

Sleep

Physicians have long believed that seven to eight hours of sleep for every individual is optimal to decrease morbidity and mortality. The duration, quality of sleep, and more recently its variability have all come into question as prognostic risk factors of disease processes.[101] This has been vividly realized in obese patients who develop obstructive sleep apnea with its airway obstruction, or those with central sleep apnea from a marginal ventilatory capacity caused by a central nervous system or neuromuscular disease. These patients develop hypertension, atrial fibrillation, dysregulated blood lipids, and insulin resistance.[102] Even shift work and daylight savings time have been implicated as disturbing sleep and creating a risk of heart attack.[103] More recently, long-term follow up of more than 20,000 participants showed than an inverted U shaped association existed between sleep duration and cognitive decline, with memory impairment resulting from sleeping less than four hours or longer than ten hours.[104] Memory impairment is the core symptom of dementia and a factor in progressing from mild cognitive decline to dementia.

With advancing age there are frequently significant changes to sleep patterns. In some cultures, afternoon napping is considered a component of a healthy lifestyle pattern, and data exist that shows it is associated with better cognitive function in some elderly populations.[105] Nevertheless, controversy exists over the optimal duration of naps with short naps (less than 30 minute) that occur frequently (four times weekly) being associated with an 84% decreased risk of developing Alzheimer's disease, while a consensus of opinion exists concerning those who nap more than two hours as more likely to show worse cognitive function.[105, 106] This subject is currently incompletely defined, but the author has noted afternoon napping by many elders over 70 years of age in the warm climates of Mediterranean Europe or South America.

Sleep is also a physiological part of what physicians know to be the circadian rhythm of the body (see regularity below). Lay people most commonly encounter circadian disturbance as jet lag. Transoceanic travel by airplane can vividly make one aware of jet lag, by awakening in the early hours of the next day or becoming markedly sleepy during the day hours of the location to where they traveled. Whereas when one is young this phenomenon is usually brief (two to four days), for the elderly the recovery time increases to seven to fourteen days. This lengthened recovery time in the author's experience occurs predominantly between 65 and 75 years of age and gives the individual a clue to his own physiological variability and aging.

Unfortunately, chronic insomnia (disturbance in sleep) is prevalent, occurring in roughly 30% of Americans and increasing in today's elderly.[107] Insomnia is characterized by difficulty falling asleep, difficulty maintaining sleep, early-morning awakening, or nonrestorative sleep.[108] It creates anxiety, daytime fatigue, and the possibility of falling asleep during the day. In the elderly it is of particular concern because it has been associated with risk of injury, cognitive impairment, depression, and an impaired quality of life. The elderly insomniacs are 2.5 to 4.5 times more likely to sustain an accident.[107] Aspects of insomnia have been linked to metabolic syndrome and cardiovascular disease, and particularly in men, difficulty in initiating sleep and nonrestorative sleep are associated with a moderately higher risk of death.[108] Insomnia's association to premature aging should be particularly concerning because of associations with mechanisms of inflammation and changes in immunity can explain our recognition of heart disease and cancer as the leading cause of deaths in men (Table 2 on page 60). One clear sign of insomnia is the bad habit of falling asleep while watching television which has been a common abnormality during the era of America's present elderly population. Other insomnia risk factors are addressed specifically for the elderly by the National Institutes of Health at: https://www.nia.nih.gov/health/good -nights-sleep. Every reader who has this problem should review the information provided on this site. A thorough discussion of the causes of insomnia are presented at: https://www.nhlbi.nih .gov/health-topics/insomnia.

In summary, normal sleep continuity is considered to be most important for the maintenance of cardiovascular and immune system functions, providing a physiological and psychological balance. Suboptimal sleep disturbs your body's regularity (circadian rhythm) and other physiological systems (hormone and the autonomic nervous system).

Regularity

Regularity is a term most often used by elderly patients to describe their bowel habits to physicians. In the simplest sense, regularity could be described as the consistency of the defecation pattern individuals experience. It is mediated by both adaptive and non-adaptive factors. We can choose when and what we eat (fasting-food cycle), how and whether we exercise, when and under what conditions we sleep, and what environment we live within. These are all adaptive factors and under an individual's control to some extent. On the other hand, the body has specific functions designed to operate on their own that are not under the conscious control of the individual. Doctors call this the circadian rhythm which the author will attempt to explain in simple terms.[109] This nonadaptive circadian rhythm is linked to a individuals' personal reserve and their comorbidities. If they have many comorbidities of important systems (e.g., the lungs, heart, and hormones) resulting in limited personal reserve, their circadian rhythm may already be impaired. This circadian rhythm is tied to releasing hormones (adrenal epinephrine and norepinephrine) when we awaken and assume the upright posture in the morning, a second elevation in the afternoon, and recession of the hormones during the depth of our sleep cycle. The circadian rhythm constantly interacts between the hormonal system and the autonomic nervous system, and can be disrupted by some comorbidities (e.g., sleep apnea) that affect both systems. The autonomic nervous system controls our heart rate, moves food along our gastrointestinal tract, controls sweating and shivering, and sends us messages when it is time to void urine or defecate.

Modern medicine knows much, but there is much still to learn in the twenty-first century (call the unknown factor X). We know that in the mid-brain hypothalamus a central master clock has the ability to reset important sub-clocks within our bodies in a twenty-four hour cycle.[109] Important sub-clocks include the hormonal system (i.e., adrenal glands and other X factors), the autonomic nervous system (innervating the heart, the sigmoid colon, the stomach and intestine, the sweat glands, and X) and an important sub-clock that the author will designate as the personal reserve sub-clock. The personal reserve sub-clock reflects the individual's physical and mental resilience and ability to cope with acute events. Individual clocks must be constantly reset as life and its activities occur, ensuring survival and synchrony between our body and the environment. Sweating in a hot environment, for example, maintains a synchrony with the internal environment (the autonomic nervous system dilating your peripheral vasculature to give off heat by dilatory activation of your blood vessels which also requires stimulating the heart for a greater cardiac output to help dissipate the heat and maintain blood pressure). Imagine the reverse scenario with entering a cold body of water, the autonomic nervous system constricts your blood vessels, slows your heart rate, and adjusts the external skin if necessary, inducing a shiver to generate heat. These changes do not call into play (to our knowledge) the hormonal endocrine system which usually needs more time to respond to an external challenge. You can imagine with the above scenarios if you have an impaired cardiac system comorbidity, your failure to respond could lead to low blood pressure with dizziness or fainting, or high blood pressure with a burden on the heart that creates a heart attack. Your personal reserve as an elder is what is threatened by comorbidities and leads to the warning signs such as those we see at tourist places in Hawaii advising elderly heart patients not to go near volcano viewing platforms. Whether such signs are directed at lung patients to avoid sulfurous gasses, or because of the heat in the area, the warning signs are clear and are urging you to know your own personal reserve.

A practical example is international air travel that affects all of the factors expressed in this lifestyle section (i.e., diet, exercise, environment and sleep), and should bring to mind a measure of your individual personal reserve in accessing your ability to recover your "normal" regularity or rhythm. In international travel from west to east, which shortens the normal sleep cycle, massive resets begin in progress. Studies have shown that exposure to light or daylight has a beneficial effect probably on the mid-brain master clock (via eye to pineal gland to unknown mechanisms and melatonin), that may help in re-establishing the normal sleep cycle. Airlines try to induce this by feeding their passenger earlier than the norm, and then awakening them for "breakfast" which is not their regular fasting-food cycle. These mechanisms are thought to promote better "staying awake" in the new environment. However, as an elder knows, jet lag lasts longer with aging (particularly after 70 years). In the author's experience, one of the last regularity factors to come back into normal wellness or personal regularity is the bowel pattern (which is mediated by the autonomic nervous system function to the sigmoid colon). During this period some studies recommend mild exercise and avoiding alcohol, but unquestionably with aging, recovery is prolonged.

To conclude this discussion of the major components of lifestyle, rest assured that there is positive evidence of long-term benefit of these recommendations. To estimate the association between healthy lifestyle and the number of years free from major diseases one may gain, a prospective study of twelve European populations (116,000 people) who were free of major noncommunicable disease (noninfectious) were examined from 1991 to 2006.[110] The number of years between ages 40 and 75 years without chronic disease, including diabetes (adult type), coronary heart disease, stroke, cancer, asthma, and COPD was examined. Examining four varying lifestyle patterns showed the highest number of disease-free years were enjoyed by those who maintained a normal weight (BMI less than 25), and at least two of the following factors: never smoking, physical activity, and moderate alcohol consumption. Comparing the best lifestyle with the worst lifestyle indicated that men gained 9.9 years and women 9.4 years of freedom from chronic diseases.[110]

Preventive Measures
Medicare preventive services

The elder citizen of the US is truly blessed thanks to policies set by the US Preventive Services Task Force (USPSTF) during the past decade to bring preventive services to the population. The USPSTF is an independent, volunteer panel of nationally recognized experts in prevention, primary care, and evidence-based medicine. The Task Force makes evidence-based recommendations about clinical preventive services to improve the health of all Americans. The Task Force comprehensively assesses the potential benefits and harms of services to prevent disease in people without signs or symptoms, including screening tests, behavioral counseling, and preventive medications. When an elder views the range of prevention services available to them, it is both surprising and humbling.(Go to https://www.cms.gov/Medicare/Prevention/PrevntionGenInfo/medicare-preventive-services/MPS-QuickReferenceChart-1.html for a full list of services.)

Most elders have not utilized the services whether from ignorance, lack of digital access or skills to access the site, or fear of medical prevention. These services, which consist initially of a face-to-face preventive physical examination, are extended to each new beneficiary during the first twelve months of Medicare enrollment. They seek to identify the leading causes of diseases in the US population and extend preventive examinations and guidance for prevention of adverse outcomes. Whereas the Task Force has created controversy within the medical community during the past decade (i.e., whether or not to recommend annual mammography or annual PSA blood tests), it has also focused on inadvertent downstream consequences within the US health care system.

The author calls attention to this latter aspect existing within the current US health care system. An incidental or new finding in a physical examination, blood study, or diagnostic test must carefully be considered within the context of the age of the patient and existing comorbidities of the patient. The physician must bear in mind the possibility of a false positive test and the existing medical error rate involved in any further investigations for that patient. Even when such examinations are indicated, both the patient and those in the medical community must reflect upon the maxim "primum non nocere" (first, do no harm).[111] As medical society groups call for "choosing wisely," elders should be aware of this perspective of the physician guiding his patients in shared decision making of the risk/benefit of all tests.[112]

Vaccines

The author believes that most elderly persons in the US have realized that the anti-vaccination campaigns, which came into the public's view in 2017 and 2018, directly led to the tragic re-emergence of measles across the US in 2018 and 2019. The US intelligence community has found that anti-vaccination groups were funded in part by foreign adversaries to sow discord in various communities throughout the US. Their mission threatens all the elderly of the US. Virtually every elder in the US should embrace (1) annual inactivated influenza vaccine for the elderly, (2) two doses of the recombinant zoster vaccine (Shingrix), and (3) the pneumococcal vaccine. Depending upon their comorbidities, they should opt for either PCV 13 alone, or PCV 13 and PPSV23 administered one year later depending on whether they have sustained a personal history of pneumonia. According to the American Heart Association (2020), recent evidence of the benefit of influenza and pneumococcal vaccine indicates adults over 50 who got flu vaccines during a hospitalization had a 28% lower risk of a heart attack the following year. They also had a 47% lower risk of a mini stroke or transient ischemic attack (TIA), 85% lower risk of cardiac arrest and 73% lower risk of overall death. These preventive measures are paramount, because they prevent or limit the adverse effects of the "normal" influenza (H3N2), prevent shingles, and lessen the probability of recurrent pulmonary pneumonias. Other vaccines exist which may be employed in special circumstances (i.e., hepatitis A or B), and currently we are seeking a solution to controlling COVID-19 in part by vaccine. As this book goes to press, two COVID-19 vaccines (mRNA vaccines of Pfizer and Moderna Pharmaceutical) are being distributed across the US, and an additional one (an adenovirus vaccine of Johnson and Johnson Pharmaceutical) became available in March 2021. Although some physicians are currently concerned during the COVID-19 pandemic that the anti-vaxxers will undermine the "herd immunity" being sought, it appears the seriousness of COVID-19 has muted the anti-vaxxers' campaigns of resistance. The appearance of coronavirus variants seems to indicate that the mutations will necessitate medical attention for more years than 2020 and 2021. We will have to follow and respond accordingly.

Medications

As previously discussed in the secondary prevention of health, medications in the last sixty years have afforded Americans an outstanding advantage over their ancestors (Figure 7 on page 31). Aspirin, statins, beta-blockers, ACE-inhibitors/ARBs, calcium antagonist drugs, all have contributed to the mitigation of heart attacks, strokes, peripheral vascular disease, kidney disease, heart failure through their effects on the heart and its vascular system. Antibiotics in suppressing bacterial infections have become so widely used that physicians now fear the development of antibiotic resistance and secondary adverse events.[48] Antiviral medications such as oseltamivir (Tamiflu), zanamivir (Relenza), and peramivir (Rapivab) have been prescribed to treat and abbreviate influenza illness, and now the COVID-19 seems somewhat responsive to such measures as assessed by early remdesivir studies.[113, 114, 115] Additionally, monoclonal antibody therapies of REGN-COV2 and LY-CoV555 have entered the antiviral arena and have shown efficacy in treating COVID-19.[116, 117] These efforts are heartening to all elders who currently are the most vulnerable to COVID-19.

The amelioration of the symptoms of benign prostatic hypertrophy, which occurs in most men at some point as they age, is facilitated preventively by the drug class of agents finasteride (Proscar) and dutasteride (Avodart), which seeks to block the effects of testosterone and mitigate the increase in interstitial tissue of the prostate volume.[118] There is also a broad array of secondary preventive medications prescribed to elderly Americans for cancer, hepatitis C, and HIV illness. These medications, which emerged during the last century, are the main reason many of today's elderly have survived, are functional, and enjoy some measure of wellness. The elder who says, "I do not want to take pills," has not been educated, does not know the facts stated above, and if recalcitrant, can suffer the grief of a morbidity that limits his/her functionality, quality of life, and can permanently impair his/her body and personal reserve.

Physical therapy
The author has observed that physical therapy following unintentional injuries or accidents renders preventive benefits, especially in men. These injuries are usually provoked by sport or leisure activities but may result from chronic osteoarthritis of the knee or hip (work or sport related). Most non-professional athletes think that they can recover on their own, rather than turning to those with the knowledge and skills in this matter. In contrast, professional athletes have already recognized the benefit of such personnel in their recovery from injuries, and they quickly follow the advice of such experts. Even without such advice and direction, elderly patients in their 70s or 80s, who have difficulty in

ambulation and function, should be aware of their limitations caused by constantly decreasing muscle mass and osteoarthritic changes associated with progressive aging. The elderly can benefit from having exercise trainers or other allied health professionals who can offer skilled physical therapy.

CHAPTER NINE

Physical Health of Elderly Men

Introduction

THIS PRIMER SEEKS to offer elderly American males in the twenty-first century a basic understanding of their individual health. It cannot present every aspect of health for all conditions. It can, however, provide the basic knowledge that each individual needs to recognize their individual risks and to choose preventive or surveillance measures going forward. They should now understand:

1. Their lifecycle and the effects imposed upon them during childhood and youth by their parents, culture, the environment, and religion.
2. What important events, personal habits, career or work-related exposures, and personal lifestyle choices during the *formative* period of their lives which have affected their existing or possible comorbidities now as an elder.
3. Their need to have a document in hand that reminds them and their care givers of their individual risk factors (family history, blood studies, and imaging data), past major system illnesses, and past surgical and injury reports.
4. Their need to have a document in hand that lists their current vaccines and medications.

These documents provided at the time of an individual health visit or crisis event will help decrease the medical error rate of 10% to 15% or more that exists in the current American medical system.[119] Unfortunately, the true medical error rate is buried (no pun intended) beneath the term "unintentional accidents" on death certificates.[119] Readers can help themselves receive better medical care by having these documents.

Finally, the author must address the masculine idea that "baby boomer" men were encouraged to emulate as adults. As children, men in the author's 80+ cohort were initially impressed as children by Tarzan movies and John Wayne Westerns or World War II films. As younger adults, we encountered new heroes like the Rambo character of the Vietnam era, and the comeback hero character of Rocky Balboa. During these *early origin* and *formative* periods of our lives there emerged a consistent model for masculinity and male behavior for the baby boomers. Society expected men to seek status, demonstrate toughness and independence, and avoid signs of effeminacy (i.e., weakness or emotion).[120] Early studies of the baby boomers' health behavior show men predominantly choose men doctors, engage in risky behaviors, avoid self-care, and do not always heed medical advice.[120] These attitudes and behaviors, of course, have contributed to the known and silent comorbidities they now experience and recognize as underlying conditions. Bear in mind that men on average can expect to die approximately five years sooner than women; they outrank women on causes of death associated with chronic diseases; and currently, early COVID-19 data show that men comprise 60% of confirmed cases and 70% to 80% of deaths.[121, 122] Unfortunately, in early COVID-19 data, people, particularly men, between the ages of 75 and 84 and those over 85 have an increased death rate of 200 times and 630 times, respectively.[122]

Suffice it to say that the current baby boomer elderly male gets sick at a younger age, develops more chronic illness, and ends up costing the health care system more.[123] While women go to the doctor more often, men ignore medical advice and prevention and ignore symptoms until they become more serious and costly. A 2000 survey by the Commonwealth Fund (https://www.commonwealthfund.org/publications/fund-reports/2000/mar/out-touch-american-men-and-health-care-system) found that three times as many men as women failed to see a doctor the previous year, and more than half of all men had not had a physical examination or a cholesterol test.[123] These traits do not bode well during the COVID-19 pandemic. Men can reshape their thinking to seek a full life with the prevention, surveillance, and wellness described herein.

Medically Observed Clues to Aging and Risks

Physicians' observations of symptoms and patients have led to some common clues of underlying maladies and pending disease states which occur predominantly with aging. Let us review some of them:

GI sphincters

GI sphincters are defined as annular muscles surrounding and able to contract or close a body opening. In the gastrointestinal tract the failure to close the opening between the esophagus and stomach leads to gastroesophageal reflux (GERD) or substernal burning that commonly arises during the night. One awakens with a "brash" of acid in the mouth, particularly after a spicy meal, excessive chocolate, or heavy alcohol intake. GERD is usually not noted until the age of 60, but it can occur earlier in those who are obese (with compression of the stomach by excessive fat). Those who experience GERD after 75 years of age may voluntarily decrease their alcohol intake to avoid this symptom.

Similarly, the anal sphincter is not important to most men (unlike women who can be affected earlier from childbirth procedures) until they begin to realize why after 75 years they need to wear underwear. Whereas flatus (bowel gas) occurs throughout life, varying in each individual, in older men, a relaxed sphincter is unable to control all colon contents, resulting in gaseous fecal staining of underwear. To compound this problem, medications can contribute to an increase of flatus in many patients. This is indicative of aging, not disease. These aging changes of the GI tract are present in 90% of elderly men observed and treated by the author.

Low back pain and baggy pants bottoms

Many of the current generation of elderly men in America engaged in relatively jarring sports and activities that sent forceful impacts throughout the spine. Progress in orthopedic medicine for fifty years has involved replacement and fixation (hips and knees), but it has not focused on prevention. Accordingly, low back pain is prevalent and a common complaint in 7% to 10% of elderly men.[124, 125] It is associated with a multiplicity of spinal osteoarthritic changes, which are often difficult to pinpoint despite x-ray and MRI investigations.[125] Nonetheless, men experience the gradual loss of height resulting from the spinal damage beginning around age 70, and their vulnerability to low back injury increases. In a practical way, they can become aware of this when the bottom of their pants begins to appear baggy (longer than normal); the shrinking of their vertebral disc spaces are placing them in danger of low back pain in the lumbar areas. Heed the warning sign. A second sign more common in those over age 80, is the preference for an SUV (generally higher from the ground) rather than the sedan or glamorous sports car of their past. Low back pain places a damper on entering and exiting those vehicles, particularly if there is an existing knee or hip comorbidity. These practical factors are common. A recent publication from British physiotherapists calls attention to a negative mindset associated with low back pain based upon myths about how to solve it.[126] They debunk common erroneous beliefs about how to solve low back pain and offer an evidence-based educational program to inform the public (www.lowbackpaincommunication.org)[126]

Decreasing lifting strength over time

Most current American elderly men grew up in the post-WWII era, a time when males commonly displayed a "macho" mentality. Strength and independence were features of a man's character. This transmitted to today's tough image of work trucks as passenger vehicles. However, subliminal messages about "being strong" challenge men when they realize that they are unable to lift as much as they did in the past. This is due to the loss of strength and muscle mass (sarcopenia to doctors), which begins to be progressive at age 65 to 70, depending on one's exercise activities and comorbidities. Despite regular training or exercise, men experience a progressive decrease of muscle strength to age 80 years, when all but few (5%?) can lift what they were accustomed to lifting when they were younger. The message here is acknowledge your loss of strength, avoid injury, and utilize assistance for heavy loads (e.g., suitcases).

Urinary frequency and nocturia

Autopsy studies show that prostate disease in the form of benign prostatic hypertrophy (BPH—a tissue increase) will start in men around the age of 30 and reach a peak prevalence of 88% in all men by age 80.[127] Genetic family history is a strong signal to men of their individual possible risk of "prostate trouble" or prostate cancer, and at what age it might occur. The need for increased frequency of urinary voiding (more than four to five times in sixteen hours of being awake) or the onset of nocturia (awakening from sleep during the night to void urine) should alert men to the possibility of prostrate trouble. A few men are able to reach 80+ years and sleep a full eight hours without urinary disturbance. On the other hand, some men who have diabetes (spilling sugar in urine) or an infection (rare bladder infection) can also develop the symptoms of frequency and nocturia. Other comorbidities such as sleep apnea contribute to urinary disturbances. Consultation with a urologist will sort out the multiple conditions that present with these symptoms. Symptoms of hesitancy (difficulty starting urination), decreased force of stream, and evidence of an enlarging prostate with bladder residual are additional important symptoms.

Proprioceptive (feeling) loss over time

The body has special fibers in the nerve endings of the feet and fingertips that feed our brain information concerning body position. Men with diabetes often encounter a neuropathy (nerve disease) that decreases the transmission of this proprioceptive information from the soles of the feet to the brain and can contribute to falls (Figure 11 on page 71). This problem can appear as early as 60 to 65 years in some diabetics depending on the overall treatment and status of their disease. On the other hand, even elders in their late 70s and definitely those in their 80s have difficulty (compared to their youth) in fastening shirt cuff links or small buttons. These tasks, which were seemingly quite normal at one time, remind us of the changes in peripheral nerves affecting a variety of sensory functions (feeling, temperature, and balance) which are increasing risks of injury with aging.

Anemia

Anemia, defined as a blood hemoglobin (Hb) below 12 g/dl in women and 13 g/dl in men is common in old age, affects an elder's physical function and is associated with increased mortality.[128] Whereas in the last century it was regarded within the medical community as a part of "normal" aging, medical science today recognizes that anemia in the elderly most commonly is caused by chronic diseases or iron deficiency.[129] These chronic diseases include the injuring process of inflammation giving rise to cancer, immunological diseases, kidney disease, and infections. [129, 130] Although aspects of aging that we do not currently fully understand (senescence cell death) may exist, every elder should be aware of their hemoglobin (Hb), which is provided in the simplest of blood tests taken as part of the preventive Medicare examination. This information can lead their physician to finding existing comorbidities of which the patient is unaware (e.g., hidden colon and rectal cancer, blood dyscrasias, and chronic kidney disease). It is an important test to survey annually by every elder. The author has found no information regarding the existence of a true "aging" anemia.

Hair loss and skin thinness over time

All elders are aware of changes in hair texture, density, and finally hair loss as they age. This again has a component of heredity but is not associated with the inherited male baldness pattern (frontal and crown), which can appear in young men in their mid to late 30s and become progressive thereafter. The further loss of hair seen from aging, with its declining level of blood testosterone, indirectly affects the scalp and leads to a change in texture (more wiry) and loss of density. These changes in hair molecules affect the melanin of the hair with follicle blanching it of color and forming the "snowbirds" (Northerners who spend winter months in the South) of our elderly communities. Physiological variation, of course, (possibly dependent on heredity) can result in thin whiteness or full hair whiteness, reminding us of the complexity of the body that we do not fully understand.

The author has been struck by skin thinness, which has appeared in the 80s. Carrying branches or other objects can, in fact, create a traumatic bruise or scar (often without symptoms) is now recognized as skin senescence or thinness. The tough skin of youth has now given way to less resilience to trauma, even without some vitamin deficiency (e.g., vitamin C deficiency) or medication interfering with the clotting mechanisms. These changes are initially unsettling, but they are part of the aging process for those over 80. Skin senescence becomes a major factor in healing after an operative procedure. Healing from any surgery, trauma, or infection must be expected to take longer than when the patient was younger. This is especially true on the forearms and lower legs where the blood flow may be impaired (from silent vascular comorbidities). The use of protective clothing (e.g. covering gloves, long pants, proper comfortable shoes, etc.) will help protect against these injuries.

Eyesight and visual changes

The author chooses not to comment on the approach each elder must make in adjusting to early visual blurring resulting from the early cataracts that occur with aging. Cataract surgery (eye and laser) evolved during the medical era of the author. It is apparent that when vision interferes with the function of reading, ambulating safely, preparing meals and the other necessities of life, each individual must choose one of those current modalities. Large ophthalmology practices in the US may offer these procedures to everyone (with Medicare insurance) at the earliest sign of cataracts; the author believes the risks involved in accepting such offers outweigh the benefits. The offer of a procedure for the sake of personal convenience goes against the author's belief in "primum non nocere" (first, do no harm). Procedures can go wrong; errors can and sometimes do happen. At 80+ years many elders can drive, read, and work safely with corrected lenses. Opting for cataract surgery must be weighed and balanced by each individual to meet his own needs with evaluating the risk/benefit outcomes for themselves.

Gingivae (gum) recession

Getting particles of food wedged between the teeth is usually a transient, albeit annoying, phenomenon during the *formative* and *transitional* periods of life. Dental care in the popular media and in televisions commercials is currently directed at enhancing "whiteness" and avoiding the yellowing of aging teeth. On occasion in today's world, prosthetic caps are made and placed to correct individual gaps and enhance a cosmetic "bright smile." Given that the latest mortality data places life expectancy in the US at 78.6 years (reflecting a decrease in recent years), it becomes difficult for elders to focus on cosmetic procedures at the end of their 70s or in their early 80s.[74] It is at this point, however, that gingiva recession from aging appears. Receding gum lines are usually localized. Dental consultation will only advise you of regular dental care, flossing carefully, and stimulating the gingiva with an electric toothbrush. The goal here is to prevent gingivitis (inflammation) by utilizing the above methods twice daily if necessary to lower the bacterial population in these areas and avoid further problems (bone loss in the area). These measures, to the author's knowledge, are the state-of-the-art treatment for this common development of gingiva recession. The author cautions against the use of the traditional wood toothpick, which is commonly available in restaurants in the Midwest, South, and Southwest, because it can injure the gingivae. If dental floss is not available, the corner of a business card made of soft paper provides a better and safer instrument.

Major Diseases in 2020 in Elderly Men

The major causes of death in men are cardiovascular disease, prostate and colon cancer, and unintentional injuries, and will be addressed in this section (Table 2 on page 60).[62] This primer cannot include all the caveats the author would like to share with the male reader, particularly for those older than 80 years. They will have to be addressed in the future. This primer is to build your health literacy to a basic level and prepare you for an overall understanding of current existing risks.

Cardiovascular diseases

Cardiovascular disease results from vascular atherosclerosis, which ultimately leads to heart attack, stroke, and peripheral artery disease, and is one of the causes of erectile and sexual dysfunction (via the penile artery). Vascular atherosclerosis is affected by both genetic factors and acquired factors as shown in Table 3 on page 62 and Figure 14 below. All American elderly men should know if their family history includes cardiovascular disease, and they should agree to obtain blood studies, which are provided at no cost by Medicare. Knowledge of their total cholesterol, HDL cholesterol, LDL cholesterol, and triglycerides is imperative to assess their risk of atherosclerosis leading to the process of heart attack and stroke. In families with a history of premature cardiovascular disease (i.e., a father less than 55

FACTORS INFLUENCING VASCULAR AGING

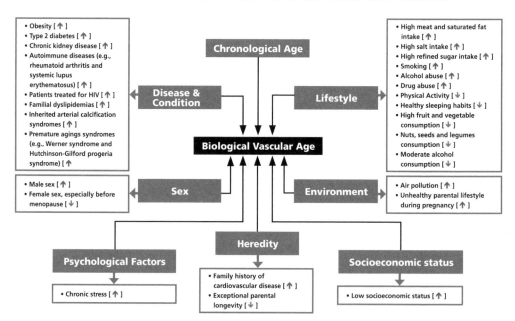

FIGURE 14. Factors influencing vascular aging . These variations account for biological variability +- 5 years. Adapted from Hamczyk MR, et al.[77]

years of age, or a mother less than 60 years of age), a lipoprotein (a) should also be obtained.[131] Additionally, the test of high sensitivity CRP is a measure of vascular inflammation, which responds in part to the effects of decreasing one's cholesterol level with the class of statin medications. The atherosclerotic process is also accelerated by such adaptive risk factors as poor diet, cigarette smoking, obesity, and a sedentary lifestyle. These risk factors can set in motion a process of inflammation which leads to atherothrombosis, tissue injury, and organ (heart, kidney, and peripheral blood vessels) damage in a long-term continuous manner during the *formative* and *transitional* periods of life until the occurrence of an event (Figure 15).[132, 133, 134] The most common consequences of these processes during life in today's elders were the occurrence of heart attacks (myocardial infarction), sudden deaths, and now today heart failure.[132, 133, 134] During the last decade the mortality rate for heart disease has decreased, but because of a 23% growth in the number of US adults over 65 years to the current fifty to sixty million, the number of deaths attributed to heart disease has increased.[27, 135]

Recent data in the US have shown a decline in life expectancy since 2006 especially for Hispanics, African Americans, and Native Americans due to social determinants of disease and the opioid crisis. COVID-19 accelerated this trend. Fortunately, the development of modern therapeutic cardiovascular interventions and medicines has markedly decreased heart attacks, sudden deaths, and strokes over the last thirty years permitting an extension of life (albeit with the presence of more heart failure), and those interventions do result in a better quality of life for today's elderly (Figures 6 and 7 on pages 30 and 31).

Cancer

Cancer is the second leading cause of death in US men. In 2020, it is estimated to have occurred in 893,000 men with 321,000 deaths in 2020 (Figure 16).[136] The occurrence (incidence) of

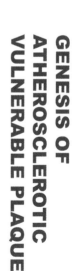

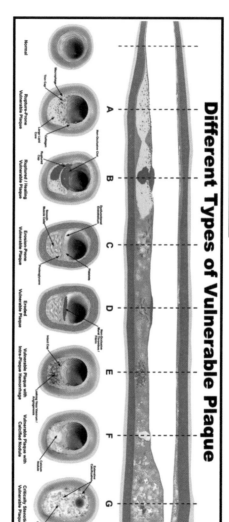

FIGURE 15. Different types of vulnerable plaque as underlying cause of acute coronary events (ACS) and sudden cardiac death (SCD). A, Rupture-prone plaque with large lipid core and thin fibrous cap infiltrated by macrophages. B, Ruptured plaque with subocclusive thrombus and early organization. C, Erosion-prone plaque with proteoglycan matrix in a smooth muscle cell-rich plaque. D, Eroded plaque with subocclusive thrombus. E, Intraplaque hemorrhage secondary to leaking vasa vasorum. F, Calcific nodule protruding into the vessel lumen. G, Chronically stenotic plaque with severe calcification, old thrombus, and eccentric lumen. Adapted from Libby P, et al.[133] and Naghavi M, et al.[134]

96

Estimated Deaths

Males			Females		
Lung & bronchus	72,500	23%	Lung & bronchus	63,220	22%
Prostate	33,330	10%	Breast	42,170	15%
Colon & rectum	28,630	9%	Colon & rectum	24,570	9%
Pancreas	24,640	8%	Pancreas	22,410	8%
Liver & intrahepatic bile duct	20,020	6%	Ovary	13,940	5%
Leukemia	13,420	4%	Uterine corpus	12,590	4%
Esophagus	13,100	4%	Liver & intrahepatic bile duct	10,140	4%
Urinary bladder	13,050	4%	Leukemia	9,680	3%
Non-Hodgkin lymphoma	11,460	4%	Non-Hodgkin lymphoma	8,480	3%
Brain & other nervous system	10,190	3%	Brain & other nervous system	7,830	3%
All Sites	321,160	100%	All Sites	285,360	100%

FIGURE 16. Estimate of projected cancer deaths in 2020. Adapted from Siegel RL, et al.[136]

cancer and deaths from cancer have been falling since 1991, but prostate, lung and bronchus, and colorectal cancers are the most common cancers in men (Figure 17).[136] Whereas prostate cancer cases occur in 21% of men, making it the leading cause of cancer, lung and bronchus cancers are the leading causes of deaths.[136] Once again genetics play an important background role. Identifying the individual with a family history of prostate or colon/rectal cancer, and changing risk factors of cigarette smoking, poor diet, and sedentary activity can lead to major prevention. Medicare preventive services from a periodic visit should identify the genetic risks, and blood studies should include the PSA. Although the US Preventive Health Services recommends against testing for PSA because of overutilization (after finding an elevated value greater than 4.0 ng/dl) in the past decade which resulted in downstream consequences of unnecessary procedures and adverse outcomes, the author urges his patients to take it. The author urges caution however, in the event of an elevated PSA result. The data must be investigated thoroughly before decisions for any interventions ensue. Elevation of PSA can occur from benign prostatic hypertrophy, infection, as well as cancer. In the current era, the examination of the prostate by MRI can be accomplished to add increased diagnostic accuracy.[137, 138] Despite most men having a concern for the development of prostate cancer, the unequivocal leading cause of cancer in both men and women is lung and bronchus in the current US elderly population (Figure 16).[136]

Moreover, as indicated previously, Medicare services provide not only wellness physician examinations and blood studies, but prostate screening, lung cancer screening with CT examinations, and colonoscopy examinations directed at the leading causes of men's cancer. It is important to access these services early in one's elderly life and obtain periodic surveillance and extended surveillance if necessary, from identified comorbidities to achieve wellness, quality of life, and that personal

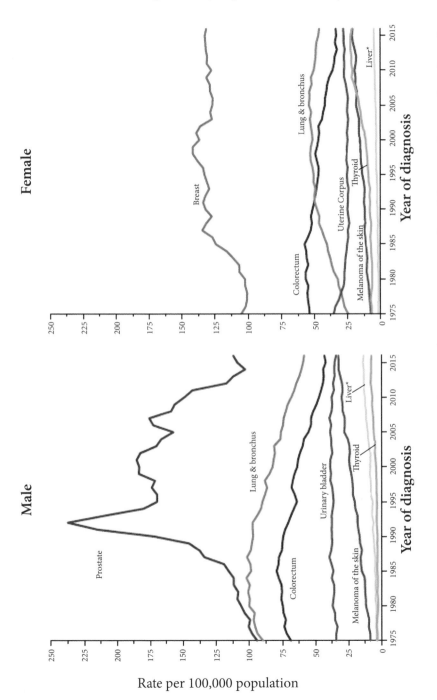

FIGURE 17. Occurrence of cancers in men and women from 1975 to 2017. Adapted from Siegel RL, et al.136from the years of 1975 to 2017. Adapted from Siegel RL, et al.[136]

resilience we all seek. Preventive services are found at: (https://www.medicare.gov/coverage/preventive-screening-services).

Unintentional injuries

The author has had the rewarding experience after the age of 65 of providing medical services predominantly to elderly patients. During this experience of more than fifteen years and before, he has realized that not only was medical prevention and surveillance very important to this population, but prevention of medical errors to this vulnerable group of patients was crucial. Whereas there had been a medical and political focus on medical errors in 2016, the data have been obscured by recent changes in the new death certificate classification codes (ICD-10) and are hidden in the 2019 data.[74, 119] Perhaps the greatest service rendered by the author to his patients was his conservative approach to every therapy by considering risks versus benefits; he also recognized the practical reality, that the medical error rate in the elderly is higher than the estimated 10% to 12% described in the past.[119] Moreover, the medical error rate was derived from in-hospital studies of Medicare patients, and did not account for the errors encountered in nursing or assisted living facilities. The author came to believe that the best way to avoid a plethora of medical errors was to provide attentive continuity of care, to keep in mind all major past medical history events, to maintain close surveillance of all comorbidities, and to be in attendance for all major therapeutic interventions. The data shown in Figure 18 best approximates the probable medical error rate which existed in 2020 (estimated 300K). Note that the number of deaths resulting from medical error exceeds that of chronic lower respiratory disease (COPD). The medical community of today currently focuses upon falls and suicide data for the elderly which seem most amenable to medical therapy, but efforts against firearm violence is also currently in today's medical and political focus.[139, 140, 141] Recent data show handguns are used in approximately three-quarters of suicides by firearms.[142]

As previously discussed in the exercise section of lifestyle, falls occur in 29% of community-dwelling elders at least once annually with 10% falling twice a year.[94] The elderly falls occur most commonly from intrinsic aging risk factors, including balance impairment (middle ear disease), visual impairment, decreased proprioception, and orthostatic hypotension (i.e., a drop in blood pressure with standing).[139] But as shown in Figure 11 on page 71, orthopedic comorbidities of curvature of the spine (osteoporosis), low back pain, and abnormalities of the hip or knee can contribute to a fall. Multiple and specific medications (i.e., sleep medicines, antidepressants, tranquilizers, and some diuretics) also play a role. To a patient who has fallen, a multifactorial assessment of the risk factors must be carried out, and interventions targeted for gait balance and strength augmentation with resolution of problems existing in the risk factor areas must be addressed.[124, 139] Whereas falls seem more consequential in women, because of the higher prevalence of osteoporosis in women, they also occur in men equally.[74] The propensity for

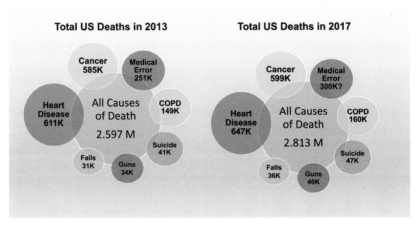

FIGURE 18. Causes of death in the US in 2013 and 2017. Adapted from Makary M, et al.[119]

fall-related harm depends on the injury on impact as well as the status of the patient. The increasingly elderly patient (i.e., older than 75 years), who encounters anticoagulation, osteoporosis, and decreasing muscle mass, is at greatest risk.

In 2020, the elder man has been identified as having the greatest risk of suicide in the elder population; men commit suicide at a rate three times that of women. Amazingly, the elderly man has twice the risk of death by suicide than dying from a fall.[74, 142] Surely, the social determinants of disease contribute to this risk and the relative lack of resilient mental health as compared to women. Whether this emanates from post-traumatic stress syndrome, status in society, economic factors, or other determinants has not been defined to the author's knowledge.

Finally, ageism and what it imposes looms in our current era as another form of unintentional injury. As discussed above it may account for more than 20% of avoidable harm in nursing facilities.[62] This is embedded unfortunately in the twenty-first century, and particularly early in the COVID-19 pandemic was demonstrated by the difficult medical triage choices made during shortages of ventilators, and the inept early medical responses in some nursing facilities.

CHAPTER TEN

Physical Health of Elderly Women

Introduction

THIS PRIMER SEEKS to offer the elderly American woman better understanding of her individual health. It cannot present every aspect of health for all conditions. It can indicate the basic knowledge all individuals must know to assess their individual risks, and then choose preventive and surveillance strategies going forward. Women must realize that data specific to their sex for more than three decades has been sparse. Medical studies and clinical trials were initially predominantly directed at males, and only in the current century has this inequity been addressed forcefully.[143] Enrollment of women and older participants in randomized clinical trials has increased over time, but women and the elderly consistently have been underrepresented. This limits a physician's ability to determine the evidence for which therapies are safe and efficacious for women.[143] Nevertheless, risk factors for elderly women have been identified (Table 5). Women should now be prepared to do the following:

1. Remember their lifecycle and the effects imposed upon them during their *early origin* period by their parents, culture, environment, diet, lifestyle, and religion.
2. Evaluate important events, personal habits, career or work-related exposures, and personal lifestyle choices that occurred during the *formative* period of their lives which

TABLE 5. Risk factors for elderly women.

Genetic risk factors	Acquired risk factors
Atherosclerosis – heart attack (coronary artery disease), stroke (cerebrovascular disease). and peripheral artery disease.	Tobacco usage – cigarette smoking
Hypertension – high blood pressure	Sedentary lifestyle – lack of exercise and activity
Hyperlipidemia – elevated cholesterol or triglycerides	Obesity
Colon cancer – colon or rectal polyps	History of preeclampsia during pregnancy
Breast cancer – hereditary breast/ovarian genes (BRCA1, BRCA2, CHEK2 and ATM)	Autoimmune disorders
Diabetes mellitus – elevated glucose or HbA1C	Frailty – unintentional weight loss, exhaustion, weakness (grip strength), slow walking speed, and low physical activity.
Osteoporosis	Against vaccines and/or preventive medications
Obesity	Belief in popular "herbal" remedies
	Alcoholism
	Substance abuse

have affected their existing or possible comorbidities now as an elder.

3. Have a document in hand that reminds them and their care givers of their individual risk factors (family history, blood studies, and imaging data), past major systemic illnesses, and past surgical and injury reports.

4. Have a document in hand that lists their current vaccines and medications.

These documents provided at the time of an individual health visit or crisis event will help decrease the widely appreciated medical error rate of 10% to 15% or more that exists in the current American medical system.[119] Unfortunately, the true medical error rate is higher. Help yourself to receive better medical care and have these documents. The author's impression is that elderly women are more likely to utilize a mobile phone than are elderly men, and he suggests that these data be entered into an App on their mobile phone for easier access in the future and to help women navigate this aspect of their health.

Medically Observed Clues to Aging and Risks

From observations of patients and their symptoms, physicians have identified some common clues that help them discover underlying maladies and pending disease states that come with aging. The author shares his observations of women aging and has sought assistance from other women's health experts. Although most clues are recognized by women, who are more sensitive than men to changes in their bodies, women tend to postpone or delay personal care due to family concerns or responsibilities for others. Let us review some of the changes women can expect to experience:

Menopausal "hot flashes"

Most women generally experience "hot flashes" during the transition period of menopause. They occur in 40% of women in the early transition and increase to 80% in the late meno-pause.[144] This frequency varies by ethnicity but sometimes persists into the elder years. One-third of women continue to have moderate or severe hot flashes for ten years after their final menstrual period.[145, 146] Usually, hot flashes persist for only four to five years, but they do create treatment challenges to avoid excess breast cancer risk. Whereas African American women report more frequent hot flashes than Caucasian women, Asian and Hispanic women have fewer symptoms.[147] Risk factors predicting such occurrence include obesity, less physical activity, smoking, race/ethnicity, and social determinants of health (lower socioeconomic status, poorer education, etc.).[148] Unfortunately, sleep disturbance can be created in as many as 60% to 70% of women and can lead to chronic insomnia.[149, 150] Therefore genetics, diet, and lifestyle all have a major impact on the pattern of hot flashes experienced by elderly women.

Treatment consists of simple measures like layering clothes, controlling the room temperature, and avoiding triggers identified by the patient. Low-dose hormonal and non-hormonal agents should be prescribed by a physician based upon risk-benefit analysis of each agent for the specific woman being treated. The complicated history of hormonal agent treatments extending back to the 1960s and the Second Women's Health Initiative randomized controlled clinical trials have provided a median follow-up of twenty years post therapy.[151] Clearly, individualized therapy using precision medicine is needed to account for genetics, race/ethnicity, existing lifestyle, cancer risks, and individual choice for this problem.

Osteopenia/Osteoporosis

Many of today's elderly women are aware of a parent or relative who had marked "curvature of the spine," and most women want to avoid such disfigurement if possible. Most American women who have insurance have obtained a bone density scan by the age of 65 years. Unfortunately, many have not. This abnormal curvature causes loss of volume in the lower third of the lung, decreasing the ability to cough effectively, and the forward position of the neck can make swallowing difficult increasing the possibility of aspiration. Risk factors for osteoporosis include family history, smoking, excessive alcohol, lack of physical exercise, early menopause, and treatments with anti-estrogens (for breast cancer) or steroids. As shown in Table 6, Medicare preventive services provide appropriate x-ray and bone density examinations as often as every two years. Fragility fractures, those that occur from low trauma, are important signs of future fractures and should prompt an evaluation for osteoporosis. Nevertheless, less than a third of women admitted to the hospital with hip fractures are referred for osteoporosis evaluation.

Fractures in the aging elderly person are associated with bone fragility. This risk between low bone mineral density (i.e. osteopenia) and the risk of fracture is continuous, and in a study of 149,524 postmenopausal women followed for one year, many more women with osteopenia than with osteoporosis (39% versus 6%) sustained fractures.[152] Contrary to popular belief propagated among women, vitamin D and calcium supplementation which can be helpful in osteopenia, is not always beneficial to stop progressive osteopenia and osteoporosis.[153]

Bisphosphonates are the first-line pharmacological treatment for severe osteopenia and post-menopausal osteoporosis. These medications reduce the risk of clinical fractures in women whose hip or spine bone mineral density (BMD) T score is less than or equal to -2.5 or who have a personal history of fragility fracture (in the hip or vertebrae).[154] Some recent data support the use of bisphosphonates in postmenopausal women with osteopenia BMD T scores of -1.0 to -2.5 who have a ten-year probability risk as calculated from the FRAX tool.[154] Moreover, a recent small study in 2019 suggests that bisphosphonates

TABLE 6. Preventive services provided by Medicare Part B.

Medicare Part B (medical insurance) Coverage
Abdominal aortic aneurysm screening
Alcohol misuse screenings & counseling
Bone mass measurements (bone density)
Cardiovascular disease screenings
Cardiovascular disease (behavioral therapy)
Cervical & vaginal cancer screening
Colorectal cancer screenings
Multi-target stool DNA tests
Screening barium enemas
Screening colonoscopies
Screening fecal occult blood tests
Screening flexible sigmoidoscopies
Depression screenings
Diabetes screenings
Diabetes self-management training
Glaucoma tests
Hepatitis B Virus (HBV) infection screening
Hepatitis C screening test
HIV screening
Lung cancer screening
Mammograms (screening)
Nutrition therapy services
Obesity screenings & counseling
One-time "Welcome to Medicare" preventive visit
Prostate cancer screenings
Sexually transmitted infections screening & counseling
Shots:
Flu shots
Hepatitis B shots
Pneumococcal shots
Tobacco use cessation counseling
Yearly "Wellness" visit

taken for a year may reduce colorectal cancer in women by 65%, but this sounds overly optimistic and requires further data.

Heavy handbag or heavy robe

The author cannot be sure when women trade a shoulder handbag (relatively large almost sac like) for a smaller handbag, or when a heavy robe gives way to a lighter version. But these changes signal the onset of decreasing muscle mass coupled with early osteopenia/osteoporosis. There are no studies that pinpoint when women make these changes, but it has been observed in many women in their 60s and early 70s. Many women will ascribe such decisions to fashion changes, but opting for lightweight clothing and lighter accessories may be a clue to physicians of possible lower limb and low back problems with insidious onset. So, women should be aware that getting rid of weighty clothes and handbags may be an early sign of declining muscle mass and underlying bone fragility that come with normal aging.

Facial and body skin changes

Today's elderly women in the US have been bombarded by messages from advertising, magazines, retail fashion companies, the beauty industry, pharmaceutical companies, and a myriad of "stay young" diets and food products that seemingly had their origin in the 1950s with the Avon Ladies to maintain a youthful appearance as long as possible. Movies and magazines reinforced this viewpoint. In the 1970s, women's magazines like *Cosmopolitan* reflected the attitudes of women's liberation and career development for women. They spoke to women who were increasingly looking for independence or a career outside of the traditional role of homemaker, and they invited women to think about romance and their own sexuality. During the last fifty years, women have been exploring a myriad of occupations offering both executive and professional positions. Concomitantly, industries emerged to support and encourage health, fitness, and the maintenance of a youthful and vigorous appearance. These changes occurred at a time when US discretionary income afforded the "luxury" of enjoying hair salons, nail salons, and day spas. Hotels added spas and salons to cater to their female clients. Such amenities were added to hotel resorts, large hotel chains, and became more commonplace. As a result, women's sports also flourished in the 1980s. Jane Fonda's workout tapes helped women in their quest for fitness and muscle tone. This fitness vogue had the positive effect of enhancing all women's sports at many levels. Articles on diet, exercise, cosmetics, herbal products, and prescription medicines to postpone or eliminate signs of aging abounded in women's magazines from *Cosmopolitan* to *Good Housekeeping.*

During this time in the medical arena, the field of plastic surgery and cosmetic interventions emerged. While opting for cosmetic surgery is an individual choice (done or for the sake of appearance), such a decision should consider age, comorbidities (e.g., poor wound healing) which may be silent, and other risks inherent in all surgical procedures. With the appearance of tanning booths, vein surgeries, and Botox (onobotulinumtoxin A) injections that temporarily relax facial muscles that cause wrinkles in the forehead and around the eyes in the last century, there emerged a new level of tolerance for individual risk one could take for the sake of beauty. Subsequently, in the twenty-first century, it is not uncommon in the US to see offers of regularly scheduled Botox injections, laser sculpting of fat removal from the stomach, hips, or buttocks, and other nasal and facial surgeries to improve one's appearance or to appear more youthful. Ageism had its effect upon the elder women of the US, who desired to defend themselves against fears associated with aging—the loss of a spouse's attention, or the threat of being replaced by a "trophy wife." These trends were created by commercial interests and the media to take advantage of the discretionary income created with the empowerment of women in their broader role in today's society.

As discussed in the men's section, the author has been struck by the changes in skin thinness which seem to appear in the 70s and 80s. In women this is especially seen with skin care products utilizing sunscreen preparations commonly used by predominantly Caucasian women in the US. Thinner and more fragile skin resulting from skin senescence and usually seen with any loss of weight, should lead women to avoid excessive sunlight (which they did not do with tanning when they were younger), and utilize protective clothing (e.g., hats, gloves, and sunscreen clothing). These preventive measures are all important to avoid aggravating skin changes that could lead to skin cancers. These changes are initially unsettling but are a part of the aging process. These vulnerability changes become a major factor in healing considerations if the patient must have any operative procedure. Healing from any surgery, trauma, or infection must be expected to be of longer duration than when they were younger. This is especially true on the forearms and lower legs where the blood flow may be impaired (from vascular comorbidities). Therefore, the use of protective clothing will help prevent such injuries.

Vulvovaginal atrophy and bladder incontinence

When women go through menopause, they experience a decrease in or loss of estrogen, and with that comes the onset of vulvae dryness, burning, itching, and sometimes pain during sexual intercourse (dyspareunia). This loss of normal secretions associated with aging and regression of tissue has been reported to affect more than 50% of older women, and previously was referred to as vulvovaginal atrophy.[155] More recently, however, specialists in the field have also associated bladder urinary frequency, urgency, and other abnormalities associated with sexual intimacy under a broader term, named Genitourinary Syndrome of Menopause. Because the urinary bladder and vagina share a close anatomical common wall, new treatments such as pelvic floor physical therapy and vaginal dilatation therapy have emerged. As estrogen declines with aging, there is a thinning of the vaginal epithelium (inner layer), reduction in lubrication, and decrease of elasticity with friability, which can lead to pain during sexual activity. The FDA has approved the use of vaginal estrogen creams and prasterone (dehydroepiandrosterone) vaginal inserts to treat the tissues directly with minimal hormonal systemic effects. An oral medication, ospemifene, has also recently been introduced and allegedly activates estrogen pathways in some tissues while blocking estrogen pathways in other tissues.[155] The long-term safety of ospemifene is not known and clinical trials are needed. The Women's Health Initiative study of 45,663 post-menopausal women using vaginal estrogen was somewhat reassuring regarding the long-term effects of vaginal estrogens.[156] Neither cardiovascular disease nor cancers were increased among women using vaginal estrogens over a median follow-up of 7.2 years.[156] Nevertheless, the fear of breast cancer and hormonal therapies of the past have affected many elderly women's wanting to avoid hormonal supplementation of any kind. Although the author has very limited data in elderly women regarding these difficulties, it is likely that these symptoms have led to an earlier loss of interest in or abandonment of sexual activity and intimacy in many women, indirectly affecting their long-term personal relationships. The beneficial data regarding the effects of these vaginal estrogens on bladder competency were examined in an exhaustive review by the Cochrane Database. It concluded there was some evidence that local estrogen vaginal creams may improve incontinence with overall reduction of one to two fewer voids in twenty-four hours; and there was less frequency and urgency.[157]

Minor adverse events of vaginal spotting, breast tenderness, and nausea occurred in some women. Nevertheless, complete data for these problems have not been systematically gathered for women, especially in the elderly, and needs further study.

Major Diseases in 2020 for Elderly Women

The major causes of death in women are cardiovascular disease, breast, lung, and colon cancer, and unintentional injuries (Table 2 on page 60).[74, 136] This primer cannot address the myriad of caveats the author wants to share with female readers, particularly for those greater than 75 years old. That will have to be addressed in the future. This primer aims to impart a basic level of health literacy and prepare older women for an overall understanding of the major risks currently existing to their health.

Cardiovascular disease

Cardiovascular disease is the leading cause of morbidity and death for women in the US and globally.[27, 158] Overall, one in three women die of cardiovascular disease, and although recognized for many years to be different than for men, sex-specific data have only been generated in the twenty-first century. Sex-related risk factors include hypertension, diabetes, hyperlipidemia, atrial fibrillation, perimenopausal hormone therapy, and psychosocial stress.[158] These factors contribute to the development of vascular atherosclerosis and endothelial dysfunction which ultimately leads to heart attack, stroke, and peripheral artery disease. Susceptibility to cardiovascular disease is affected by both genetic factors and acquired factors as shown in Table 5 on page 104. All American elderly women should know their family history of cardiovascular disease and should have blood studies done, which are provided at no cost by Medicare. Early or premature atherosclerosis is said to occur when family history reveals a father less than 55 years of age, or a mother less than 60 years of age who sustained a cardiovascular event (heart attack or stroke). Knowledge of their total cholesterol, HDL cholesterol, LDL cholesterol, triglycerides and hsCRP (high-sensitive CRP) is imperative to assess their risk of atherosclerosis leading to heart attack or stroke. Women's individual risk seems accelerated following menopause; their vascular disease is different from men and manifest in more diverse ways. In addition to obstructive coronary artery disease, their lesion is most commonly an erosion rather than a ruptured plaque; and women also sustain spontaneous coronary artery dissection (Figure 15 on page 96).

Uniquely, women sustain stress-induced cardiomyopathy (Takotsubo disease), and microvascular coronary artery dysfunction with endothelial dysfunction more frequently than men.[159] Adverse pregnancy outcomes during life have also been associated with later risk of cardiovascular disease events.[158] Specifically, low birthweight infants, eclampsia, pre-eclampsia, and gestational diabetes should serve as warning signs of potential for cardiovascular disease and to lead to a plan for prevention. In a national cohort of approximately 50,000 women, pre-term delivery was a strong independent risk factor for ischemic heart disease that waned over time but remained substantially elevated up to forty years later.[160]

During the last twenty years, physicians have become aware of the fact that women do not always sustain the same symptoms of a heart attack experienced in men (chest pressure or pain radiating to the left arm or jaw), but may present atypical signs of shortness of breath, back or abdominal pain, and unexplained nausea.[161] Women are more prone to the development of a stroke because they frequently leave hypertension untreated, which causes an internal stiffness of their heart muscle (diastolic dysfunction) leading to atrial fibrillation. Women have about a 20% to 30% higher risk of stroke than men with atrial fibrillation.[158] Whereas many of these comorbidities occur somewhat silently after menopause, knowledge of their presence with aging can help avoid their bad outcomes.

Cancer

Cancer is the second leading cause of death in US women and was estimated to have occurred in 912,930 women with 285,360 deaths in 2020 (Figure 16 on page 97).[136] Although the incidence of cancer and deaths from cancer have been falling since the early 1990s, lung and bronchus, breast, and colorectal cancers dominate in women (Figure 17 on page 99).[136] In 2020, an estimated 276,489 breast cancer cases occurred, but the largest number of deaths in women occurred from lung and bronchus cancers (Figure 16).[136] Women rarely forget a family history, which often leads to early detection. Since genetics does play a major role in breast cancer, knowing the family's history of the disease leads to screening blood biomarkers and mammography, and if cancer is detected, advances in medical pharmaceutical therapy prevent death. Today's recent data indicate that breast cancers account for 30% of all cancers in women, and although it is the most frequent women's cancer, it is not the leading cause of death in women (Figure 16).[136] With more women smoking, especially since the 1960s, and fifty years of medical progress against breast cancer, including prevention medications like tamoxifen and raloxifene, lung cancers have become the major cause of death in US women (Figure 16). Whereas an increase in smoking patterns emerged in women born around the 1960s answers some of the cause, more recent evidence of the impact of pharmaceutical primary prevention medications (e.g., tamoxifen and raloxifene) have also contributed to this more favorable outcome for breast cancer.[162] Randomized trials have shown that taking tamoxifen for five years reduces breast cancer risk for twenty years.[163] Nevertheless, women in general in the US (especially after the history of the early hormonal fears during the controversial early menopausal treatment era), are reluctant to adopt preventive therapies.[164] Thus, health education about this preventive benefit is lacking and essential.

Similarly, the author has encountered an entrenched reluctance in many elderly women to undergo a colonoscopy examination to prevent colorectal cancers despite the evidence of its effectiveness. Most colorectal cancers arise from colon polyps that progress from being small to large (greater than 8 mm). This progression in polyp size changes it to becoming cancerous and is estimated on average to occur over ten years in those at average risk.[165] The recommendation for preventive colonoscopy was made in general for those over 50 years of age, but a family history of polyps or colon cancer may impact this decision. Those with a family history of polyps or colon cancer should be examined at an earlier age. In 2020, the US Preventive Task Force issued specific recommendations for those elders aged 76 to 85 years based upon their precise family history and comorbidities.

With recent alternative detection investigations becoming more available (e.g., Cologuard stool samples or MRI colonoscopies), it seems that a better acceptance by women of this preventive measure will occur in the coming years.

Unintentional injury

Preventing unintentional injury of women is challenging. Many of the causes are similar to men, but to the author, women appear to be more susceptible to trying new diets and new herbal supplements that are offered up in the marketplace. Most women commonly seek medical advice when they perceive a problem, but they could benefit from prevention and surveillance to discover unknown harms and to avoid medical errors. Consider this case encountered by the author.

Vignette Case

———————————⁑———————————

The 44-year-old woman was active, apparently healthy, and engaged in family activities. She had sustained a gallbladder operation (cholecystectomy) at age 38 years for gallbladder sludge (cholestasis) and had no other major medical abnormalities. In the 1980s, she pursued physical fitness and beauty through various weight-loss diets. She began taking an eclectic group of mixtures but eventually adopted the "grapefruit diet," which stringently required eating only grapefruit for a month. After two weeks, the patient developed the onset of chronic abdominal "deep" aching. During the third week of the diet, acute abdominal pain forced a visit to the emergency room of the local hospital. Evaluation disclosed evidence of acute pancreatitis. During hospital evaluation, the patient was discovered to have a pancreatic divisum, a common congenital pancreatic anomaly, occurring in approximately 10% of individuals. Whereas 95% of such persons are asymptomatic, fewer than 5% have infrequent bouts of pancreatobiliary-type pain or develop mild pancreatitis. This was a silent potential comorbidity unknown to the patient most of her life.

Gastroenterologists opined that the stringent grapefruit diet had led to the precipitation of the biliary and pancreatic symptoms. She was ordered to stop all extreme diets and follow a standard bland diet. All symptoms abated without recurrence. Subsequently, over the next thirty years, no recurrence of abdominal symptoms occurred. Evidence data concerning the "grapefruit diet" was never collected to the author's knowledge.

The author has had the rewarding experience after the age of 65 of providing medical services predominantly to the elderly. During this experience of more than fifteen years and before, he has realized that medical prevention and surveillance are very important to this population, and prevention of medical errors is especially important for this vulnerable group of patients. Whereas there had been a medical and political focus on medical errors in 2016, the data have been obscured by recent changes in the new death certificate classification codes (ICD-10) and are hidden in the 2019 data.[74, 119] Perhaps the greatest service rendered by the author to his patients was his conservative approach to every therapy by considering risks versus benefits; he also recognized the practical reality that the medical error rate in the elderly is higher than the estimated 10% to 12% described in the past.[119] Moreover, the medical error rate was derived from in-hospital studies of Medicare patients and did not account for the errors encountered in nursing or assisted living facilities. The author came to believe that an approach of attentive continuity of care, considering all major past medical history events, keeping close surveillance of all comorbidities, and being in attendance for all major therapeutic interventions resulted in a plethora of medical errors being avoided. The data shown in Figure 18 on page 101 best approximates the probable medical error rate which existed in 2020 (estimated 300K). Note that the number of deaths resulting from medical error exceeds that of chronic lower respiratory disease (COPD). The medical community currently focuses upon falls and suicide data for the elderly which seem most amenable to medical therapy, but efforts against firearm violence is also currently in today's medical and political focus.[139, 140, 141] Recent data show handguns were used in approximately three-quarters of suicides by firearms.[142] Moreover, in the latest death data, deaths resulting from the use of legal or illegal drugs rose at double the age-adjusted rate for unintentional injuries.[74] This finding has accounted for the recent interest in "opioid abuse news" prevalent during 2019 and 2020.

CHAPTER ELEVEN

Psycho-Social Determinants of Disease

Introduction

AFTER A DISCUSSION of the overall health of both men and women, encompassing prevention, surveillance, and wellness within the perspective of their existing comorbidities, it is appropriate to examine those societal factors which influence peace of mind and the quality of life of elders in the US (Figure 8 on page 45). The concept of **social determinants of disease** has only emerged into a broader view in US society in the twenty-first century.[55, 56, 57] The World Health Organization defines social determinants of disease as "the conditions in which people are born, grow, work, live, age, and the wider set of forces and systems shaping the conditions of daily life." [166] These determinants include income, social status, and education, environmental factors (including safe drinking water and clean air), healthy workplaces, safe housing, health-promoting communities and roads, safe employment and working conditions, social support networks, and access to healthcare.[167] These non-medical factors all contribute to the current political discussions on health inequality that exist in impoverished communities throughout the US.

Health inequality has emerged both politically (championed by the progressive movement) and within the health care arena (as a matter of population health). Discussion of health inequality has primarily focused on why Americans have worse health outcomes than their counterparts in other high-income countries.[168] It raises a key question: How can the United States spend

$9,169.00 per capita versus an average of $8,402.00 per capita in comparable countries (twenty-seven European Union countries) and have worse outcomes? The US is an outlier in social spending for the elderly ($6522.00/capita) as compared to the European Union ($4,268.00/capita).[168] Social spending on elders in the US, even with its positive effects, may be too little, too late to reverse the deleterious effects incurred in the *early origin* period or *formative* periods of life that resulted in comorbidities and an unhealthful lifestyle. That in effect is why health literacy at an early stage is so important and should be available to every citizen in the US.[11]

The relationship between social spending by the government in the US and the population it serves is a major topic in the current political discourse. A call to support the younger and working-age population (e.g., health care insurance, education, parental leave, child allowances, and unemployment benefits) is at the very heart of the "progressive movement." We US elders must realize that our educational and socioeconomic level have affected our overall health through the indirect effects of culture, religion, environment, and lifestyle over a lifetime. The effects of these social determinants cannot be denied and bear directly on cardiovascular and other diseases which are the leading cause of death in the US.[169, 170]

In the United States, "We the people" are the source of power, and, according to the US constitution, the government must reciprocally "preserve, protect and defend."[171] Nevertheless, COVID-19 has unequivocally exposed that the healthcare system does not provide equality of treatment for the most vulnerable citizens. African Americans, Latinos, and indigenous Native Americans are dying disproportionately during the COVID-19 pandemic.[171] The poor, the forgotten in rural areas, and those without the benefit of insurance are suffering in this pandemic from health inequities that exist widely across the nation.[171]

From this population perspective, the author will now focus more on the individual elder and aspects of economic peace of mind, security, safety, and a personal psycho-social community that affect an elder's health.

Economic Peace of Mind

As an individual passes through the arcade of life, many changes ensue. In the transition period of life, more often than one would desire, many individuals experience a serious illness, divorce, or an economic setback that has influenced their economic well-being as an elder. Despite the urging of commercial and government forces for workers to establish a retirement plan and not to depend only upon social security for income as an elder, only about 50% of Americans have a supplemental retirement income plan, according to the most recent data.[172] Saving for retirement has not been easy for many of today's elders, who have been affected by a) the growing income inequality of the last thirty years, b) the financial crisis of 2007-2008, and c) the COVID-19 pandemic that began unfolding in 2020 (Figure 19A and B).

When today's elders became 62 to 65 years old in the year 2000, they had achieved a slow growth of savings (despite income inequality which was in progress) that peaked in 2007, only to be depressed markedly by the year 2010 (Figure 19A).[172] Many considered part of the middle class fell into poverty and had to utilize any savings that existed in a retirement plan. The rise of the digital age led to job loss for some, and having to master new technologies to become employable made finding a new job difficult. Many individuals could not afford to retire. The digital age required knowledge and computer skills for which their level of education had not prepared them (Figure 19B). The elder often accepted jobs with lower income and reduced benefits to supplement any social security to which they

Most families—even those approaching retirement—have little or no retirement savings

Median retirement account savings of families by age, 1989–2016 (2016 dollars)

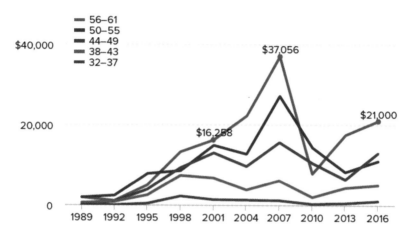

Legend:
- 56–61
- 50–55
- 44–49
- 38–43
- 32–37

$40,000

$37,056

$21,000

20,000

$16,258

0

1989 1992 1995 1998 2001 2004 2007 2010 2013 2016

Note: Scale changed for visibility. Retirement account savings include funds in 401(k)-style defined contribution plans and in IRAs.

FIGURE 19A. Retirement savings of families by age from 1989 to 2016. Adapted from Morrissey M[172].

were entitled. This cascade of events now added to COVID-19 indicates the ongoing further threat of economic insecurity now facing America's elderly.

Economic peace of mind, the author would opine, means having the ability to meet one's daily needs—the food, shelter, and hopefully the lifestyle they were accustomed to during their good working years. In the US, elders are encouraged to "downsize" which means moving to a smaller dwelling, eliminating excess belongings, and getting accustomed to living with less. Downsizing has become the model for elderly retirement. With increasing income inequality, more and more elders are forced

College-educated families have much larger retirement account balances

Median savings for families age 32–61 with retirement savings by education, 1989–2016 (2016 dollars)

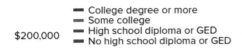
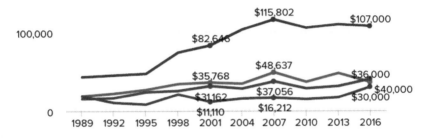

Note: Retirement account savings include funds in 401(k)-style defined contribution plans and in IRAs. "College degree" includes associate degrees.

FIGURE 19B. Importance of education in 2020 on retirement accounts. Adapted from Morrissey M[172].

to distinguish their wants from necessities. Many elders have been able to accomplish this goal, but far too many have not. The past practice of keeping the elderly parents in the child's home, has given way to a change in family values and the proliferation of nursing homes and assisted living facilities for the elderly, all demanding financial resources. Most of today's elders realize that they are "on their own" and worry whether they will outlive their income and savings[4] All elders must plan for these factors by making an ongoing assessment of their health and economic needs. It is because of these adverse factors in the twenty-first century that the progressive movement in the US political arena argues for some form of health care for all, secure social security that escapes a poverty level, and a clean environment.

Safety and Security

An individual's peace of mind is not only threatened by the economics of his or her existence, but also by the safety and security of the environment. This is especially true after the age of 75 years, when comorbidities appear with increasing frequency and threaten the strength of one's mobility and individual physical capacities, with increasing osteoarthritis and loss of physical strength (declining muscle mass with aging). In the US, these aspects of the aging process can make elders feel vulnerable and threatened by crime and gun violence in many cities, simply from the aging process. Unfortunately, even though only 1% of the US population of approximately 330 million people may engage in criminal behavior, given the tolerance of gun violence by many political leaders, those three million people pose an imminent threat to the well-being of all elders.[173, 174] The World Health Organization mortality data found that Americans are twenty-five times more likely to be victims of a gun-related murder and eight times more likely to die by firearm suicide than people in other developed countries.[175] This unfortunate truth must be acknowledged when elders seek a safe environment. These factors in part have led to the development of safe elderly communities in Florida and Arizona, where gated security or enhanced protection measures for elders are provided. Housing with wider corridors, more bathroom safety designs, and with meal and delivery services have also been developed. Obviously, this alternative is not available to many elders because of income inequality. This is a national problem that each elder must plan for individually.

Further threats emerge during elders' mid-70 years, when approximately 70% will experience the emergence of a major comorbidity or a major disease event. Depending on their access to competent medical care and treatment, ongoing health care surveillance or extended surveillance, and chronic preventive follow up, many can and will return to a good quality of life. Nonetheless as discussed previously in lifestyle regularity of personal reserve, at age 75 years there is an acceleration of the rate of loss of muscle, with changes in type I muscle fibers and muscle atrophy, changes in endocrine hormones that secondarily affect muscle loss, and recognition of chronic diseases which impose ongoing inflammation.[176] At this age, medication dosages often have to be adjusted (usually decreased) due to changes in enzyme metabolism systems, decrease in kidney function, less muscle mass metabolism, and vulnerabilities (e.g., skin thinness) not previously evident. This age-related physiological decline unfortunately encourages the onset of **frailty** which is the antithesis and opposite of one's personal reserve. What is frailty?

At one time, frailty was recognized and defined by the following clinical features: unintended weight loss, loss of strength, low levels of activity, poor endurance, or fatigue, and slowed performance (Figure 20).[176] The presence of three of these factors identified patients at increased risk of poor health outcomes, falls, poor functional outcomes in daily living, hospitalizations, and early deaths. Frailty was most commonly associated with symptomatic long-term disease, decline in function, and decreased post-operative survival. Gradually with investigative studies it has become recognized that with continued aging these processes are associated with many poor operative outcomes, increased use of health care resources and institutionalization, cognitive decline, disability, and mortality.[177] Currently, frailty is conceptualized as a multidimensional clinical condition related to progressive aging with loss of physiological and psychological systems in an elder's personal reserve, resulting in less ability to cope with the daily stress of life and illness.[178] Today frailty is estimated to be present in 16% of

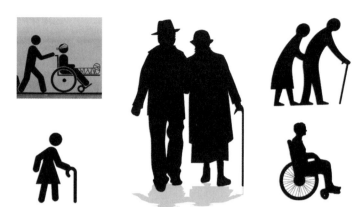

FIGURE 20. Frailty of unintended weight loss, low activity, loss of strength, poor endurance, fatigue, and slowed performance.

community-dwelling elders and is most prevalent in women.[177] Nonetheless, women tolerate frailty better than men with lower mortality rates at any frailty level or age. Among the best practical interventions to delay or reverse frailty is a Mediterranean diet with strength training and protein supplementation. Those interventions ranked highest in relative effectiveness and ease of implementation.[82, 177] The lack of comprehensive care for frail elderly people within the current dysfunctional health care system of the US has been identified and demands available affordable health clinical care, home health care services, and a plan by a multidisciplinary team.[179] Organizations have emerged to bring focus upon this elder problem, but recommendations generally fall to a low priority in political ad¬ministrations (http://medcaring.org).[180]

Finally, and amazingly not included in the current definition of frailty, but in every elder's mind is the looming possibility of cognitive decline with the threat of dementia or worse, Alzheimer's disease, with their aging.[4, 75] This condition limits ambulation and activity and imparts a pathway to frailty. The most current Global Burden of Disease study of neurological disorders in the US shows that stroke, Alzheimer's disease and other dementias, and migraine over the last thirty-five years are the dominant neurological diseases in the US.[181] These data show that the conditions of stroke have decreased, while Alzheimer's and other dementias, as well as migraine have remained steady (relatively unchanging) during this period. Amazingly there is a marked difference of incidence and disability (1.2-fold to 7.5-fold) of all neurological diseases across the geographic states of the US.[181] This threat looms silently in the back of the minds of many elders who have relatives or ancestors that they perceive have sustained either dementia or Alzheimer's disease. These factors should be discussed openly with the health care physician when they are present. There are medical diagnostic and therapeutic solutions to clarify these threats.

Personal Psycho-Social Environment

In reality, the "messy" lives of today's elders of the baby boomer generation have been complicated by war, international tension, and diseases that have become global in scale. In one form or another, they have seen and been emotionally involved in the conflicts in Korea, Cuba's Bay of Pigs, Viet Nam, Bosnia, Afghanistan, Iraq, and Syria. Looming in the background, impressed in their minds from the school drills of the 1950s and 1960s, was the possibility of a nuclear war. These geopolitical threats now seem diminished in 2020, when compared to the global threat of the COVID-19 pandemic, which has claimed the lives of many elderly in a silent stealth-like manner. Some US states have reached the alarming conclusion that the elderly are expendable; their political decisions prioritize the well-being of the economy, now facing two years of recession, over the well-being of older Americans. Notwithstanding that reality, the components discussed below are important components that the author has observed in those elderly who survive such trials.

Community

The community in which elders live life presents the reality of their economic situation, safety, and security in a daily fashion. The "blue zones" that are said to exist on earth do not usually paint us a mental picture of a gloom and doom environment but suggest the elements of a desirable climate with brightness, fresh air, clean water, beautiful nature, and low stress (a personal determination). While one elder may seek bustling activity, another may seek the tranquility of relative silence as we have seen in the lives of well-known artists (e.g., Georgia O'Keefe in New Mexico or Claude Monet in Giverny). Nevertheless, there are common features. In Ikaria, Greece, the environment of the Cycladic islands presents a physical environment that provides this safe and secure almost idyllic vision. Surely some Americans see the canyons of Arizona or Utah or the golf courses of Florida and California in this manner. But within Ikaria is a sense of shared responsibility for every person in the community. The community comes together in regular periodic fashion for common decisions that affect all as town halls or celebrations, or to address an external accident or threat to one of its members. Community labor accomplishes collective harvesting and other common chores for the benefit of all. This ingrained behavior in part emanated from the Greek culture of eons past for survival upon such isolated islands. They live modestly, in a healthy way, sharing simple pleasures, and supporting their friends, families, and those living in the community alone. This is what US baby boomers are seeking either in our existing urban settings, a second home (perhaps downsized), or even an assisted living facility. Unfortunately, the "John boy" culture depicted in the 1970s television show, *The Waltons,* has passed us, and income inequality over three decades has resulted in families needing two workers to make ends meet. Today's image of children caring for their parents into old age is vanishing from the US. Few elders in the US enjoy this lingering twentieth-century family retirement insurance.

Elders need what doctors look for to benefit their patients—a support system. Is the patient safe and secure? How impaired are they with their comorbidities? Do they have caring family members or friends nearby in their personal sphere? Who helps them oversee their health needs? Are they engaged in society, or are they lonely or possibly suicidal? Establishing a socially engaged community in which the elder can live and interact is vitally important to most elders.

Personal companionship

Most humans benefit from having companionship in their lives, and this is especially true of elders. Companionship refers to having company, friendship, or being with someone in a friendly way in a sustained manner. Companionship may come from their spouse, an alternative spouse (to a widow or widower), a lover, an intermittent friend, a community in a cloister (monastery or convent), or a pet animal. A friend is usually a person other than a family member, spouse, or lover whose company one enjoys and for whom one feels affection. A vast amount of medical data indicates true companionship, in one form or another, confers health benefits, improves the quality of life, and decreases morbidity and mortality.[182]

When a married couple survives together to their 70s, they have endured a multitude of tests throughout life that have prepared them to support each other for the trials of aging. The very presence of a spouse provides conversation, social engagement, physical nurturing (see below), security during an illness, emotional support for adverse events, and "two minds are better than one" for life-changing decisions. Their personalities and harmony have made them endure together whatever life threw at them. Some psychologists call attention to their ability to create fair compromises: each partner identifies the closely held dreams and values of the other that they cannot (or should not) negotiate, and finds some way to concede. They cuddle and touch each other physically with affection, not just eroticism .[183] Depending upon their lifestyle as previously discussed, they may physically endure in mutual contented harmony for an additional fifteen to twenty years together as elders.

In contrast, the death of a spouse not only brings grief and loss, but a complete alteration of the lifestyle of the surviving elder widow or widower. Many seek to marry again or find an alternative spouse, seeking to replace the same attributes they enjoyed in their previous life, but it is complicated. The elder baby boomer is frequently physically fit with personal reserve, sexually interested into their early 80s, and adrift in a second life that may last ten or more years. The digital era has offered them opportunities for meeting younger brides or male companions, engaging in social networks for the elderly, and finding a companion from among a remaining pool of eligible widows or widowers who were friends in the past. These choices have been tempered by their appraisal of their individual health, their fears or paranoia about their individual economic resources, the expectations of their children and family, and a myriad of self-doubts about their own capacities to re-engage in an intimate relationship with another person. Many choose to simply emulate the grandparents of the twentieth century and remain a single elder. These factors are poignantly portrayed in the Netflix movie *Our Souls at Night,* starring Jane Fonda and Robert Redford. The movie highlights the loneliness that ensues in the everyday life of a widow or widower, the relative decrease of social engagement, and the loss of physical nurturing that comes from a companion. The physical nurturing of intimately sleeping with someone (with or without sexual activity), holding them, caressing them, or receiving their warmth and smell imparts physical and physiological contentment to both the sleep pattern of the individual and their physiological body. This movie brings into focus the difficulty of losing intimacy and companionship as an elder and the constraints many elders face because of social obligations from their earlier life. It gives elders much to ponder.

The author has experienced and believes that this close association sometimes is achieved with a dutiful pet animal who is a listener (sometimes with a response), a friend during exercise, and a guardian at night. The pet's proximity to the elder as a constant presence reassures the frail, who may not feel safe and secure. Their physical contact in many ways send messages of affection and caring to the elder. Often, they are a committed servant. In the author's view, this particular form of companionship seems to please many widows.

The virtues of cloister living have been confined in the past to religious orders for centuries. These persons pursued dedication to prayer, community works, and a tranquil environment. This monastic view presented itself in usually more idyllic settings to permit inner reflection and religious prayer. Today a variation of this phenomena in the US has also emerged among elders past the age of 80. With less mobility, the concerns of safety and security expressed above, and less desire to travel, a segment of society is reshaping some assisted living communities in urban areas. These communities are on the elders' "home ground" where they have spent the majority of their lives. Such cloisters bring together long-time friends who share similar political and societal views, interests, religious interests, and pastimes. Card playing groups, book clubs, cultural gatherings, and local sport teams, offer a sense of community they are familiar with and more easily embrace. Whether this will persist with the younger elders of the baby boomer group, who are more aggressive, remains to be determined.

In the 2020s, society across the US has come to recognize the gay and lesbian community. These individuals, who have existed for all of recorded history (since Classical Greece) and sustained some of the worst aspects of the social determinants of disease, now enjoy the right to marry, have families, and become elderly together. The author cannot comment directly upon the specific health problems of this group of patients beyond the HIV disease and its control, but within the next decade, more will be known based on medical data derived from this group. It appears to the author that the benefits and trials of all married couples will be found in this community, i.e., they will share the same benefits, morbidities, and mortality described in this primer. A curious feature of this community is how often single elder women (divorced, widowed, or over a lifetime) choose a female companion (usually a lady friend) in their elder years. The author has no knowledge of the physical nurturing of this relationship but realizes there is little suicide in this group of elders.[74] In contrast, the elder man does not fare well. The risk of suicide is reported to be three times that of women.[74] This difference, as previously mentioned, seems rooted in the social determinants of disease that overwhelm men at the end of life. Nevertheless, the loss of companionship in a crisis is akin to removing affection and love at a crucial time to the elder man. Unfortunately, the data support this viewpoint.[182]

PART III.

CONCLUDING REMARKS

Conclusion

THE PERSONAL CAVEATS that physicians offer to address specific health situations are beyond the scope of this primer. A basis for health literacy must be established taking into account the current level of knowledge in today's elderly population.. As the baby boomers complete their entry into the elderly by 2030, their medical knowledge will undoubtedly be greater than that of 2020 elders. After experiencing the ramifications of the 2020 geopolitical and economic cycle and the changes brought about in the public health sector from COVID-19, the author has hope for a more global perspective of solutions directed at both the climate crisis and global public health. The need for more global planning in global cooperative organizations is apparent. The author also looks forward to preparing a more patient-focused individual text in the near future that is directed at an improved and available US healthcare system that is progressive and equitable with improved benefits that address the social determinants of disease.[171]

The digital world offers usable wearable health technology employing diagnostic and therapeutic applications with artificial intelligence in a manner to guide both prevention and surveillance of individual patients.[52] It can offer smartphone access (through mobile Apps) to permit ready availability of the elder's individual genetic, medical, vaccination, and medication records. The smartphone provides a vehicle following clinical "aging at home" therapies and facilitates assessment of health care outcomes. These data portend epidemiological studies that will benefit society in innumerable ways. The coming decade promises an amazing array of possibilities to provide improved health care for the elderly throughout the digital world.

References

1. He W, Goodkind D, Kowal P. U.S. Census Bureau International population reports—an aging world 2015. Report no. P95/16-1. Washington, DC: Government Publishing Office, 2016. http://www.fiapinternacional.org/wp-content/uploads/2016/10/An-Aging-World-2015.pdf

2. Dzau VJ, Inouye SK, Rowe JW, Finkelman E, Yamada T. Enabling healthful aging for all—the National Academy of Medicine grand challenge in healthy longevity. *N Engl J Med*. 2019;381(18):1699-1701. doi:10.1056/NEJMp1912298

3. US Census Bureau. Projected age groups and sex composition of the population: main projections series for the United States, 2017-2060. Washington, D.C.: US Census Bureau. Population Division, 2018.

4. Carstensen LL. We need a major redesign of life. *The Washington Post*. November 29, 2019. https://www.washingtonpost.com/opinions/we-need-a-major-redesign-of-life/2019/11/29/a63daab2-1086-11ea-9cd7-a1becbc82f5e_story.html

5. Fried LP, Rowe JW. Health in Aging—Past, present, and future. *N Engl J Med* 2020; 383(14):1293-96. doi:10.1056/NEJMp2016814

6. Pizzo PA. A prescription for longevity in the 21st century: renewing purpose, building and sustaining social engagement, and embracing a positive lifestyle. *JAMA*. 2020;323(5):415-416. doi:10.1001/jama.2019.21087

7. Mayberry LS, Schildcrout JS, Wallston KA, et al. Health literacy and 1-year mortality: mechanisms of association in adults hospitalized for cardiovascular disease. *Mayo Clin Proc*. 2018;93(12):1728-1738. doi:10.1016/j.mayocp.2018.07.024

8. Williams MV, Baker DW, Parker RM, Nurss JR. Relationship of functional health literacy to patients' knowledge of their chronic disease. A study of patients with hypertension and diabetes. *Arch Intern Med*. 1998;158(2):166-172. doi:10.1001/archinte.158.2.166

9. Glicksman E. Health illiteracy is nothing new in America. But the pandemic magnifies how troubling it is. *The Washington Post*. August 2, 2020. https://www.washingtonpost.com/health/health-illiteracy-is-nothing-new

-in-america-but-the-pandemic-magnifies-how-troubling-it-is/2020/07/31/09 1c8a18-d053-11ea-9038-af089b63ac21_story.html

10. World Health Organization. Health Literacy. www.who.int/healthpromo tion/conferences/9gchp/health-literacy/en.

11. Climie R, Fuster V, Empana J-P. Health literacy and primordial prevention in childhood—An opportunity to reduce the burden of cardiovascular disease. *JAMA Cardiol.* 2020 Jul 29.doi:10.1001/jamacardio.20202864. Published online ahead of print.

12. UnitedHealthGroup. Health literacy key to better health outcomes. www .uhg.com/health-literacy-research.

13. Fanaroff AC, Califf RM, Harrington RA, et al. Randomized trials versus common sense and clinical observation. *J Am Coll Cardiol.* 2020;76(5):580-589. doi:10.1016/j.jacc.2020.05.069

14. US Census Bureau. https://www.census.gov/library/publications/2011 /compendia/statab/131ed/population.html

15. Thomson B, Emberson J, Peto R, et al. Childhood smoking, adult cessation, and cardiovascular mortality: Prospective study of 390 000 US adults. *J Am Heart Assoc.* 20 Nov 3;9(21):e018431. doi.org/10.1161/JAHA.120.018431

16. Agustí A, Hogg JC. Update on the pathogenesis of chronic obstructive pulmonary disease. *N Engl J Med.* 2019;381(13):1248-1256. doi:10.1056/ NEJMra1900475

17. Celli BR, Wedzicha JA. Update on clinical aspects of chronic obstructive pulmonary disease. *N Engl J Med.* 2019;381(13):1257-1266. doi:10.1056/ NEJMra1900500

18. Bui DS, Lodge CJ, Burgess JA, et al. Childhood predictors of lung function trajectories and future COPD risk: a prospective cohort study from the first to the sixth decade of life. *Lancet Respir Med.* 2018;6(7):535-544. doi:10.1016/S2213-2600(18)30100-0

19. Lelieveld J, Pozzer A, Pöschl U, Fnais M, Haines A, Münzel T. Loss of life expectancy from air pollution compared to other risk factors: a worldwide perspective. *Cardiovasc Res.* 2020;116(11):1910-1917. doi:10.1093/cvr/ cvaa025

20. Groh CA, Vittinghoff E, Benjamin EJ, Dupuis J, Marcus GM. Childhood Tobacco Smoke Exposure and Risk of Atrial Fibrillation in Adulthood. *J Am Coll Cardiol.* 2019;74(13):1658-1664. doi:10.1016/j.jacc.2019.07.060

21. Miller M. The Decade in retirement: Wealthy Americans moved further ahead. *The New York Times.* December 14, 2019. https://www.nytimes .com/2019/12/14/business/retirement-social-security-recession.html

22. Segal, GZ. Warren Buffett wants young people to know: Ignoring this is like 'leaving a car out in hailstorms.' *CNBC.* https://www.cnbc.com/2019/04/12 /billionaire-warren-buffett-greatest-advice-to-millennials-the-1-thing-in -life-you-need-to-prioritize.html

23. Mahmood SS, Levy D, Vasan RS, Wang TJ. The Framingham Heart Study and the epidemiology of cardiovascular disease: a historical perspective. *Lancet.* 2014;383(9921):999-1008. doi:10.1016/S0140-6736(13)61752-3

24. Dawber TR, Meadors GF, Moore FE Jr. Epidemiological approaches to heart disease: the Framingham Study. *Am J Public Health Nations Health.* 1951;41(3):279-286. doi:10.2105/ajph.41.3.279

25. Levine GN, Keaney JF Jr, Vita JA. Cholesterol reduction in cardiovascular disease. Clinical benefits and possible mechanisms. *N Engl J Med.* 1995;332(8):512-521. doi:10.1056/NEJM199502233320807

26. Joseph P, Leong D, McKee M, et al. Reducing the global burden of cardiovascular disease, Part 1: the epidemiology and risk factors. *Circ Res.* 2017;121(6):677-694. doi:10.1161/CIRCRESAHA.117.308903

27. Roth GA, Mensah GA, Johnson CO, et al. Global Burden of Cardiovascular Diseases and Risk Factors, 1990-2019. *J Am Coll Cardiol.* 2020 Dec 22;76(25):2982-3021. doi:10.1016/j.jacc.2020.11.010

28. World Health Organization. WHO global NCD action plan 2013-2020. Geneva, Switzerland: WHO. 2013. https://www.who.int/publications/i/item/9789241506236

29. Woolf SH, Schoomaker H. Life expectancy and mortality rates in the united states, 1959-2017. *JAMA.* 2019;322(20):1996-2016. doi:10.1001/jama.2019.16932

30. Chetty R, Stepner M, Abraham S, et al. The association between income and life expectancy in the united states, 2001-2014 [published correction appears in *JAMA.* 2017 Jan 3;317(1):90]. *JAMA.* 2016;315(16):1750-1766. doi:10.1001/jama.2016.4226

31. Acharya T, Aspelund T, Jonasson TF, et al. Association of unrecognized myocardial infarction with long-term outcomes in community-dwelling older adults: the ICELAND MI Study. *JAMA Cardiol.* 2018;3(11):1101-1106. doi:10.1001/jamacardio.2018.3285

32. Schelbert EB, Iyer AM, Miller CA. Detecting the prevalent vulnerable phenotype of unrecognized myocardial infarction: another benefit of CMR stress testing. *J Am Coll Cardiol.* 2020 Aug 25;76(8):958-960. doi: 10.1016/j.jacc.2020.07.004. PMID: 32819470.

33. Vähätalo JH, Huikuri HV, Holmström LTA, et al. Association of silent myocardial infarction and sudden cardiac death. *JAMA Cardiol.* 2019;4(8):796-802. doi:10.1001/jamacardio.2019.2210

34. Roberts WC. Frequency of left ventricular scars at autopsy in persons dying suddenly of coronary artery disease with or without earlier myocardial infarction. *JAMA Cardiol.* 2019;4(8):802-803. doi:10.1001/jamacardio.2019.2238

35. Messerli FH. This day 50 years ago. *N Engl J Med.* 1995;332(15):1038-1039. doi:10.1056/NEJM199504133321518

36. Dustan HP, Schneckloth RE, Corcoran AC, Page IH. The effectiveness of long-term treatment of malignant hypertension. *Circulation.* 1958;18(4 Part 1):644-651. doi:10.1161/01.cir.18.4.644

37. Wang C, Yuan Y, Zheng M, et al. Association of age of onset of hypertension with cardiovascular diseases and mortality. *J Am Coll Cardiol.* 2020;75(23):2921-2930. doi:10.1016/j.jacc.2020.04.038

38. Siling L, Schwartz JE, Shimbo D, et al. Estimated prevalence of masked asleep hypertension in US adults. *JAMA Cardiol.* 2020 Oct 28;e205212. doi:10.1001/jamacardio.2020.5212. Online ahead of print.

39. Collins R, Bowman L, Landray M, Peto R. The magic of randomization versus the myth of real-world evidence. *N Engl J Med.* 2020;382(7):674-678. doi:10.1056/NEJMsb1901642

40. King G. Health care reform and the Medicare program. *Health Aff (Millwood).* 1994;13(5):39-43. doi:10.1377/hlthaff.13.5.39

41. Kramer AM. Health care for elderly persons--myths and realities. *N Engl J Med.* 1995;332(15):1027-1029. doi:10.1056/NEJM199504133321511

42. Affordable Care Act. https://www.hhs.gov/healthcare/about-the-aca/index.html

43. Bell SK, Delbanco T, Elmore JG, et al. Frequency and types of patient-reported errors in electronic health record ambulatory care notes. *JAMA Netw Open.* 2020;3(6):e205867. Published 2020 Jun 1. doi:10.1001/jamanetworkopen.2020.5867

44. Singh H, Meyer AND, Thomas EJ. The frequency of diagnostic errors in outpatient care: estimations from three large observational studies involving US adult populations. *BMJ Qual Saf.* 2014;23(9):727-731. doi:10.1136/bmjqs-2013-002627

45. Dalen JE, Alpert JS. Concierge medicine is here and growing!! *Am J Med.* 2017;130(8):880-881. doi:10.1016/j.amjmed.2017.03.031

46. Serna DC. Lifestyle medicine in a concierge practice: my journey. *Am J Lifestyle Med.* 2019;13(4):367-370. Published 2019 Jan 7. doi:10.1177/1559827618821865

47. Ho V, Metcalfe L, Dark C, et al. Comparing utilization and costs of care in freestanding emergency departments, hospital emergency departments, and urgent care centers. *Ann Emerg Med.* 2017;70(6):846-857.e3. doi:10.1016/j.annemergmed.2016.12.006

48. Incze MA, Redberg RF, Katz MH. Overprescription in urgent care clinics—the fast and the spurious. *JAMA Intern Med.* 2018;178(9):1269-1270. doi:10.1001/jamainternmed.2018.1628

49. Greenland P, Hassan S. Precision preventive medicine—ready for prime time? *JAMA Intern Med.* 2019;179(5):605-606. doi:10.1001/jamainternmed.2019.0142

50. Rodgers GP, Collins FS. Precision nutrition—the answer to "what to eat to stay healthy". *JAMA*. 2020;324(8):735-736. doi:10.1001/jama.2020.13601

51. Centers for Disease Control and Prevention (CDC), health and economic costs of chronic diseases. Updated March 23, 2020. Accessed August 5, 2020. https://www.cdc.gov/chronicdisease/about/costs/index.htm

52. Sim I. Mobile devices and health. *N Engl J Med*. 2019;381(10):956-968. doi:10.1056/NEJMra1806949

53. Perez MV, Mahaffey KW, Hedlin H, et al. Large-scale assessment of a Smartwatch to identify atrial fibrillation. *N Engl J Med* 2019;381:1909-1917. doi:10/1056/NEJMoa1901183

54. Campion EW, Jarcho JA. Watched by Apple. *N Engl J Med* 2019;381(20): 1964-1965. doi: 10/1056/NEJMe1913980.

55. Silverstein M, Hsu HE, Bell A. Addressing social determinants to improve population health: the balance between clinical care and public health [published online ahead of print, 2019 Dec 2]. *JAMA*. 2019;10.1001 /jama.2019.18055. doi:10.1001/jama.2019.18055

56. Braveman P, Egerter S, Williams DR. The social determinants of health: coming of age. *Annu Rev Public Health*. 2011;32:381-398. doi:10.1146/ annurev-publhealth-031210-101218

57. Figueroa JF, Frakt AB, Jha AK. Addressing social determinants of health: time for a polysocial risk score. *JAMA*. 2020;323(16):1553-1554. doi:10.1001/ jama.2020.2436

58. Officer A, de la Fuente-Núñez V. A global campaign to combat ageism. *Bull World Health Organ*. 2018;96(4):295-296. doi:10.2471/BLT.17.202424

59. Nash P, Schnarrs PW. Coronavirus shows how ageism is harmful to health of older adults. *The Conversation*. June 15, 2020. https://theconver sation.com/coronavirus-shows-how-ageism-is-harmful-to-health-of-older -adults-138249

60. DePills L. Baby boomers are taking on ageism—and losing. *The Washington Post*. August 4, 2016. https://www.washingtonpost.com/lifestyle/magazine /baby-boomers-are-taking-on-ageism--and-losing/2016/08/03/43d6664c -120c-11e6-8967-7ac733c56f12_story.html

61. Malani P, Kullgren J, Solway E, et al. *National Poll of Healthy Aging: everyday ageism and health. 2020 July 13;* University of Michigan. http://hdl .handle.net/2027.42/156038.

62. Kohn NA. The pandemic exposed a painful truth: America doesn't care about old people. *The Washington Post*. May 8, 2020. https://www .washingtonpost.com/outlook/nursing-home-coronavirus-discrimination- elderly-deaths/2020/05/07/751fc464-8fb7-11ea-9e23-6914ee410a5f_story. html

63. Berger ZD, Brito JP, Ospina NS, et al. Patient centered diagnosis: sharing diagnostic decisions with patients in clinical practice. *BMJ* 2017;359:j4218. doi:10.1136/bmj.j4218.

64. Forman DE, de Lemos JA, Shaw LF, et al. Cardiovascular biomarkers and imaging in older adults. *J Am Coll Cardiol.* 2020;76(13):1577-1594. doi: 10/1016/j.jacc.2020.07.055

65. Mahmoud AN, Gad MM, Elgendy AY, Elgendy IY, Bavry AA. Efficacy and safety of aspirin for primary prevention of cardiovascular events: a meta-analysis and trial sequential analysis of randomized controlled trials. *Eur Heart J.* 2019;40(7):607-617. doi:10.1093/eurheartj/ehy813

66. Valgimigli M. The remarkable story of a wonder drug, which now comes to an end in the primary prevention setting: say bye-bye to aspirin!. *Eur Heart J.* 2019;40(7):618-620. doi:10.1093/eurheartj/ehy872

67. Peters AT, Mutharasan RK. Aspirin for prevention of cardiovascular disease. *JAMA.* 2020;323(7):676. doi:10.1001/jama.2019.18425

68. Bosetti C, Santucci C, Gallus S, Martinetti M, La Vecchia C. Aspirin and the risk of colorectal and other digestive tract cancers: an updated meta-analysis through 2019. *Ann Oncol.* 2020;31(5):558-568. doi:10.1016/j.annonc.2020.02.012

69. Huang WY, Saver JL, Yi-Ling W, et al. Frequency of intracranial hemorrhage with low-dose aspirin in individuals without symptomatic cardiovascular disease. A systematic review and meta-analysis. *JAMA Neurol.* 2019;76(8):906-914. doi: 10.1001/jamaneurol.2019.1120. Online ahead of print.

70. Orkaby AR, Driver JA, Ho YL, et al. Association of statin use with all-cause and cardiovascular mortality in US veterans 75 years and older [published correction appears in *JAMA.* 2020 Oct 13;324(14):1468]. *JAMA.* 2020;324(1):68-78. doi:10.1001/jama.2020.7848

71. Nanna MG, Peterson ED. Translating the secondary prevention therapeutic boom into action. *JAMA Cardiol.* 2020;5(2):215-216. doi:10.1001/jamacardio.2019.4959

72. US Preventive Task Force. High-priority evidence gaps for clinical preventive services. Ninth Annual Report to Congress. November 2019. https://www.uspreventiveservicestaskforce.org/uspstf/about-uspstf/reports-congress/ninth-annual-report-congress-high-priority-evidence-gaps-clinical-preventive-services

73. de Koning HJ, van der Aalst CM, de Jong PA, et al. Reduced lung-cancer mortality with volume CT screening in a randomized trial. *N Engl J Med.* 2020;382(6):503-513. doi:10.1056/NEJMoa1911793

74. Kochanek KD, Murphy SL, Xu J, Arias E. Deaths: final data for 2017. *Natl Vital Stat Rep.* 2019;68(9):1-77.

75. Lourida I, Hannon E, Littlejohns TJ, et al. Association of lifestyle and genetic risk with incidence of dementia [published online ahead of print, 2019 Jul 14]. *JAMA*. 2019;322(5):430-437. doi:10.1001/jama.2019.9879

76. Roeckelein JE. Sheldon's type theory. In: Roeckelein JE, *Dictionary of Theories, Laws, and Concepts in Psychology*. Greenwood Press; 1998:427-8.

77. Hamczyk MR, Nevado RM, Barettino A, Fuster V, Andrés V. Biological versus chronological aging: JACC focus seminar. *J Am Coll Cardiol*. 2020;75(8):919-930. doi:10.1016/j.jacc.2019.11.062

78. Kolber MR, Scrimshaw C. Family history of cardiovascular disease. *Can Fam Physician*. 2014;60(11):1016–1022.

79. American Heart Association Nutrition Committee, Lichtenstein AH, Appel LJ, et al. Diet and lifestyle recommendations revision 2006: a scientific statement from the American Heart Association Nutrition Committee [published correction appears in *Circulation*. 2006 Dec 5;114(23):e629] [published correction appears in *Circulation*. 2006 Jul 4;114(1):e27].*Circulation*. 2006;114(1):82-96. doi:10.1161/CIRCULATIONAHA.106.176158

80. Knopman DS. Mediterranean diet and late-life cognitive impairment: a taste of benefit. *JAMA*. 2009;302(6):686-687. doi:10.1001/jama.2009.1149

81. Knoops KT, de Groot LC, Kromhout D, et al. Mediterranean diet, lifestyle factors, and 10-year mortality in elderly European men and women: the HALE project. *JAMA*. 2004;292(12):1433-1439. doi:10.1001/jama.292.12.1433

82. Voelker R. The Mediterranean diet's fight against frailty. *JAMA*. 2018;319(19):1971-1972. doi:10.1001/jama.2018.3653

83. Guasch-Ferré M, Liu G, Li Y, et al. Olive oil consumption and cardiovascular risk in U.S. adults. *J Am Coll Cardiol*. 2020;75(15):1729-1739. doi:10.1016/j.jacc.2020.02.036

84. Barnad ND, Alwarith J, Rembert E, et al. A Mediterranean diet and low-fat vegan diet to improve body weight and cardiometabolic risk factors: A randomized, cross-over trial. *J Am Coll Nutr*. 2021;1-13. doi: 10.1080/07315724.2020.1869625. Online ahead of print.

85. Bao Y, Han J, Hu FB, et al. Association of nut consumption with total and cause-specific mortality. *N Engl J Med*. 2013;369(21):2001-2011. doi:10.1056/NEJMoa1307352

86. Ros E. Eat nuts, live longer. *J Am Coll Cardiol* 2017;70(20):2533-2535. doi: 10.1016/j.jacc.2017.09.1082

87. Li J, Lee DH, Hu J, et al. Dietary inflammatory potential and risk of cardiovascular disease among men and women in the U.S. *J Am Coll Cardiol*. 2020;76(19):2181-2193. doi: 10.1016/j.jacc.2020.09.535

88. Estruch R, Scanella E, Lamuela-Raventós RM. Ideal dietary patterns and foods to prevent cardiovascular disease. *J Am Coll Cardiol*. 2020;76(19):2194-2196. Doi: 10.1016/j.jacc.2020.09.575.

89. Dehghan M, Mente A, Rangarajan S, et al. Association of egg intake with blood lipids, cardiovascular disease, and mortality in 177,000 people in 50 countries. *Am J Clin Nutr.* 2020;111(4):795-803. doi:10.1093/ajcn/nqz348

90. Piercy KL, Troiano RP, Ballard RM, et al. The physical activity guidelines for Americans. *JAMA.* 2018;320(19):2020-2028. doi:10.1001/jama.2018.14854

91. Joseph G, Marott JL, Torp-Pederson C, et al. Dose response association between level of physical activity and mortality in normal, elevated, and high blood pressure. *Hypertension.* 2019;74(6):1307-1315. doi:10.1161/HYPERTENSIONAHA.119.13786

92. Li F, Harmer P, Fisher KJ, et al. Tai Chi and fall reductions in older adults: a randomized controlled trial. *J Gerontol A Biol Sci Med Sci.* 2005;60(2):187-194. doi:10.1093/gerona/60.2.187

93. Stamatakis E, Gale J, Bauman A, Ekelund U, Hamer M, Ding D. Sitting time, physical activity, and risk of mortality in adults [published correction appears in *J Am Coll Cardiol.* 2019 Jun 4;73(21):2789]. *J Am Coll Cardiol.* 2019;73(16):2062-2072. doi:10.1016/j.jacc.2019.02.031

94. Ganz DA, Latham NK. Prevention of falls in community-dwelling older adults. *N Engl J Med.* 2020;382(8):734-743. doi:10.1056/NEJMcp1903252

95. Bhasin S, Gill TM, Reuben DB, et al. A randomized trial of a multifactorial strategy to prevent serious fall injuries. *N Engl J Med.* 2020;383(2):129-140. doi:10.1056/NEJMoa2002183

96. Yu T. Yang style Tai Chi fundamentals for health professionals and instructors. https://taichihealth.com/video/tai-chi-fundamentals-for-health-professionals/

97. Kim K, Choi S, Hwang SE, et al. Changes in exercise frequency and cardiovascular outcomes in older adults. *Eur Heart J.* 2020;41(15):1490-1499. doi:10.1093/eurheartj/ehz768

98. Elliott AD, Linz D, Mishima R, et al. Association between physical activity and risk of incident arrhythmias in 402 406 individuals: evidence from the UK Biobank cohort. *Eur Heart J.* 2020;41(15):1479-1486. doi:10.1093/eurheartj/ehz897

99. Nattel S. Physical activity and atrial fibrillation risk: it's complicated; and sex is critical. *Eur Heart J.* 2020;41(15):1487-1489. doi:10.1093/eurheartj/ehz906

100. Wang Y, Nie J, Ferrari G, et al. Association of physical activity intensity with mortality. A national cohort study of 403 681 US adults. *JAMA Intern Med.* 2021;181(2):203-211. doi: 10.1001/jamainternmed.2020.6331

101. Huang T, Mariani S, Redline S. Sleep irregularity and risk of cardiovascular events: the multi-ethnic study of atherosclerosis. *J Am Coll Cardiol.* 2020;75(9):991-999. doi:10.1016/j.jacc.2019.12.054

102. Veasey SC, Rosen IM. Obstructive sleep apnea in adults. *N Engl J Med.* 2019;380(15):1442-1449. doi:10.1056/NEJMcp1816152

103. Manfredini R, Fabbian F, De Giorgi A, et al. Daylight saving time and myocardial infarction: should we be worried? A review of the evidence. *Eur Rev Med Pharmacol Sci*. 2018;22(3):750-755. doi:10.26355/eurrev_201802_14306

104. Ma Y, Liang L, Zheng F, Shi L, Zhong B, Xie W. Association between sleep duration and cognitive decline. *JAMA Netw Open*. 2020;3(9):e2013573. Published 2020 Sep 21. doi:10.1001/jamanetworkopen.2020.13573

105. Cai H, Su N, Li W, et al. Relationship between afternoon napping and cognitive function in the ageing Chinese population. *General Psychiatry* 2021;34(1):e100361. doi: 10.1136/gpsych-2020-100361

106. Asada T, Motonaga T, Yamagata Z, et al. Associations between retrospectively recalled napping behavior and later development of Alzheimer's disease: Association with APOE genotypes. *Sleep* 2020;23(5):629-634.

107. Roth T. Insomnia: definition, prevalence, etiology, and consequences. *J Clin Sleep Med*. 2007;3(5 Suppl):S7-S10.

108. Li Y, Zhang X, Winkelman JW, et al. Association between insomnia symptoms and mortality: a prospective study of U.S. men. *Circulation*. 2014;129(7):737-746. doi:10.1161/CIRCULATIONAHA.113.004500

109. Van Laake LW, Lüscher TF, Young ME. The circadian clock in cardiovascular regulation and disease: Lessons from the Nobel Prize in Physiology or Medicine 2017. *Eur Heart J*. 2018;39(24):2326-2329. doi:10.1093/eurheartj/ehx775

110. Nyberg ST, Singh-Manoux A, Pentti J, et al. Association of healthy lifestyle with years lived without major chronic diseases. *JAMA Intern Med*. 2020;180(5):760-768. doi:10.1001/jamainternmed.2020.0618

111. Rothberg MB. The $50 000 physical. *JAMA*. 2020;323(17):1682-1683. doi:10.1001/jama.2020.2866

112. Rich EC. Barriers to choosing wisely® in primary care: It's not just about "the money". *J Gen Intern Med*. 2017;32(2):140-142. doi:10.1007/s11606-016-3916-7

113. Grein J, Ohmagari N, Shin D, et al. Compassionate use of remdesivir for patients with severe covid-19. *N Engl J Med*. 2020;382(24):2327-2336. doi:10.1056/NEJMoa2007016

114. Goldman JD, Lye DCB, Hui DS, et al. Remdesivir for 5 or 10 days in patients with severe Covid-19. *N Engl J Med* 2020;383:1827-1837. doi: 10.1056/NEJMoa2015301

115. Beigel JH, Tomashek KM, Dodd LE. Remdesivir for the treatment of covid-19 - preliminary report. Reply. *N Engl J Med*. 2020;383(10):994. doi:10.1056/NEJMc2022236

116. Chen P, Nirula A, Heller B, et al. SARS-CoV-2 neutralizing antibody LY-CoV555 in outpatients with Covid-19. *N Engl J Med* 2021;384(3):229-237. doi: 10.1056/NEJMoa2029849

117. Weinrich DM, Sivapalasingam S, Norton T, et al. REGN-COV2, a neutralizing antibody cocktail, in outpatients with Covid-19. *N Engl J Med* 2021;384(3):238-251. doi: 10.1056/NEJMoa2035002

118. Unnikrishnan R, Almassi N, Fareed K. Benign prostatic hyperplasia: Evaluation and medical management in primary care. *Cleve Clin J Med.* 2017;84(1):53-64. doi:10.3949/ccjm.84a.16008

119. Makary MA, Daniel M. Medical error—the third leading cause of death in the US. *BMJ.* 2016;353:i2139. Published 2016 May 3. doi:10.1136/bmj.i2139

120. Himmelstein MS, Sanchez DT. Masculinity in the doctor's office: Masculinity, gendered doctor preference and doctor-patient communication. *Prev Med.* 2016;84:34-40. doi:10.1016/j.ypmed.2015.12.008

121. Mooney C, Kaplan S, Kim MJ. The coronavirus is killing far more men than women. *The Washington Post.* March 19, 2020. https://www.washington post.com/climate-environment/2020/03/19/coronavirus-kills-more -men-than-women/

122. Koh HK, Geller AC, VanderWeele TJ. Deaths from COVID-19. *JAMA* 2021;325(2):133-134. doi: 10.1001/jama.2020.25381. Published online 17 December 2020.

123. Cimons M. Many men avoid doctors. That can be dangerous, even deadly, for them. *The Washington Post.* April 12, 2020. https://www.washingtonpost .com/health/many-men-avoid-doctors-that-can-be-dangerous-even-deadly -for-them/2020/04/10/ffab50d0-7824-11ea-a130-df573469f094_story.html

124. GBD 2016 Disease and Injury Incidence and Prevalence Collaborators. Global, regional, and national incidence, prevalence, and years lived with disability for 328 diseases and injuries for 195 countries, 1990-2016: a systematic analysis for the Global Burden of Disease Study 2016 [published correction appears in *Lancet.* 2017 Oct 28;390(10106):e38]. *Lancet.* 2017;390(10100):1211-1259. doi:10.1016/S0140-6736(17)32154-2

125. Hartvigsen J, Hancock MJ, Kongsted A, et al. What low back pain is and why we need to pay attention. *Lancet.* 2018;391(10137):2356-2367. doi:10.1016/S0140-6736(18)30480-X

126. O'Sullivan PB, Caneiro JP, O'Sullivan K, et al. Back to basics: 10 facts every person should know about back pain. *Br J Sports Med.* 2020;54(12):698-699. doi:10.1136/bjsports-2019-101611

127. Berry SJ, Coffey DS, Walsh PC, Ewing LL. The development of human benign prostatic hyperplasia with age. *J Urol.* 1984;132(3):474-479. doi:10.1016/s0022-5347(17)49698-4

128. Penninx BW, Pahor M, Woodman RC, Guralnik JM. Anemia in old age is associated with increased mortality and hospitalization. *J Gerontol A Biol Sci Med Sci.* 2006;61(5):474-479. doi:10.1093/gerona/61.5.474

129. Weiss G, Goodnough LT. Anemia of chronic disease. *N Engl J Med.* 2005;352(10):1011-1023. doi:10.1056/NEJMra041809

130. Ganz T. Anemia of Inflammation. *N Engl J Med*. 2019;381(12):1148-1157. doi:10.1056/NEJMra1804281

131. Mehta A, Virani SS, Ayers CR, et al. Lipoprotein(a) and family history predict cardiovascular disease risk. *J Am Coll Cardiol*. 2020;76(7):781-793. doi:10.1016/j.jacc.2020.06.040

132. Dzau VJ, Antman EM, Black HR, et al. The cardiovascular disease continuum validated: clinical evidence of improved patient outcomes: part I: Pathophysiology and clinical trial evidence (risk factors through stable coronary artery disease). *Circulation*. 2006;114(25):2850-2870. doi:10.1161/CIRCULATIONAHA.106.655688

133. Libby P, Ridker PM, Maseri A. Inflammation and atherosclerosis. *Circulation* 2002;105(9):1135-1143. doi: 10.1161/hc0902.104353

134. Naghavi M, Libby P, Falk E, et al. From vulnerable plaque to vulnerable patient. A call for new definitions and risk assessment strategies: Part I. *Circulation* 2003;108(14):1664-1672. doi: 0.1161/01.CIR.0000087480.94275.97

135. Sidney S, Go AS, Jaffe MG, Solomon MD, Ambrosy AP, Rana JS. Association between aging of the US population and heart disease mortality from 2011 to 2017. *JAMA Cardiol*. 2019;4(12):1280-1286. doi:10.1001/jamacardio.2019.4187

136. Siegel RL, Miller KD, Jemal A. Cancer statistics, 2020. *CA Cancer J Clin*. 2020;70(1):7-30. doi:10.3322/caac.21590

137. Eldred-Evans D, Burak P, Connor MJ, et al. Population-based prostate cancer screening with magnetic resonance imaging or ultrasonography. The IP1-PROSTAGRAM study. *JAMA Oncol*. 2021 Feb 11. doi: 10.1001/jamaoncol.2020.7456. Online ahead of print.

138. Lee SI, O'Shea A. Community-based screening for prostate cancer. A role for magnetic resonance imaging? *JAMA Oncol*. Published online 11 February 2021. doi: 10.1001/jamaoncol.2020.7294

139. Guirguis-Blake JM, Michael YL, Perdue LA, et al. Interventions to prevent falls in older adults. Updated evidence report and systematic review for the US Preventive Services Task Force. *JAMA* 2018; 319(16):1705-1716. doi: 10.1001/jama2017.21962

140. Butler EK, Boveng HM, Harruff RC, et al. Risk of suicide, homicide, and unintentional firearm deaths in the home. *JAMA Intern Med*. 2020;180(6):909-911. doi:10.1001/jamainternmed.2020.0806

141. Maa J, Darzi A. Firearm injuries and violence prevention—the potential power of a surgeon general's report. *N Engl J Med*. 2018;379(5):408-410. doi:10.1056/NEJMp1803295

142. Studdert DM, Zhang Y, Swanson SA, et al. Handgun ownership and suicide in California. *N Engl J Med*. 2020;382(23):2220-2229. doi:10.1056/NEJMsa1916744

143. Khan SU, Khan MZ, Raghu Subramanian C, et al. Participation of women and older participants in randomized clinical trials of lipid-lowering therapies: a systematic review. *JAMA Netw Open.* 2020;3(5):e205202. Published 2020 May 1. doi:10.1001/jamanetworkopen.2020.5202

144. Santen RJ, Loprinzi CL, Casper RF. Menopausal hot flashes. *UpToDate.* https://www.uptodate.com/contents/menopausal-hot-flashes/print?topicRef=7428&source=see_link accessed current June 2020.

145. Freeman EW, Sammel MD, Sanders RJ. Risk of long-term hot flashes after natural menopause: evidence from the Penn Ovarian Aging Study cohort. *Menopause.* 2014;21(9):924-932. doi:10.1097/GME.0000000000000196

146. Tepper PG, Brooks MM, Randolph JF Jr, et al. Characterizing the trajectories of vasomotor symptoms across the menopausal transition. *Menopause.* 2016;23(10):1067-1074. doi:10.1097/GME.0000000000000676

147. Gold EB, Sternfeld B, Kelsey JL, et al. Relation of demographic and lifestyle factors to symptoms in a multi-racial/ethnic population of women 40-55 years of age. *Am J Epidemiol.* 2000;152(5):463-473. doi:10.1093/aje/152.5.463

148. Gold EB, Colvin A, Avis N, et al. Longitudinal analysis of the association between vasomotor symptoms and race/ethnicity across the menopausal transition: study of women's health across the nation. *Am J Public Health.* 2006;96(7):1226-1235. doi:10.2105/AJPH.2005.066936

149. Ohayon MM. Severe hot flashes are associated with chronic insomnia. *Arch Intern Med.* 2006;166(12):1262-1268. doi:10.1001/archinte.166.12.1262

150. de Zambotti M, Colrain IM, Javitz HS, Baker FC. Magnitude of the impact of hot flashes on sleep in perimenopausal women. *Fertil Steril.* 2014;102(6):1708-15.e1. doi:10.1016/j.fertnstert.2014.08.016

151. Minami CA, Freedman RA. Menopausal hormone therapy and long-term breast cancer risk: further data from the women's health initiative trials. *JAMA.* 2020;324(4):347-349. doi:10.1001/jama.2020.9620

152. Siris ES, Chen YT, Abbott TA, et al. Bone mineral density thresholds for pharmacological intervention to prevent fractures. *Arch Intern Med.* 2004;164(10):1108-1112. doi:10.1001/archinte.164.10.1108

153. Khosla S, Melton LJ 3rd. Clinical practice. Osteopenia. *N Engl J Med.* 2007;356(22):2293-2300. doi:10.1056/NEJMcp070341

154. Ensrud KE, Crandall CJ. Bisphosphonates for Postmenopausal Osteoporosis [published online ahead of print, 2019 Oct 17]. *JAMA.* 2019;10.1001/jama.2019.15781. doi:10.1001/jama.2019.15781

155. Crandall CJ. Treatment of vulvovaginal atrophy [published online ahead of print, 2019 Sep 26]. *JAMA.* 2019;10.1001/jama.2019.15100. doi:10.1001/jama.2019.15100

156. Crandall CJ, Hovey KM, Andrews CA, et al. Breast cancer, endometrial cancer, and cardiovascular events in participants who used vaginal

estrogen in the Women's Health Initiative Observational Study. *Menopause.* 2018;25(1):11-20. doi:10.1097/GME.0000000000000956

157. Cody JD, Jacobs ML, Richardson K, et al. Oestrogen therapy for urinary incontinence in post-menopausal women (review). *Cochrane Database of Systematic Reviews.* 2012;10:1-99. doi:10.1002/14651858.CD001405.pub3.

158. Cho L, Davis M, Elgendy I, et al. Summary of updated recommendations for primary prevention of cardiovascular disease in women: JACC State-of-the-Art Review. *J Am Coll Cardiol.* 2020;75(20):2602-2618. doi:10.1016/j.jacc.2020.03.060

159. Mendirichaga R, Jacobs AK. Sex differences in ischemic heart disease—the paradox persists. *JAMA Cardiol.* 2020;5(7):754-756. doi:10.1001/jamacardio.2020.0819

160. Crump C, Sundquist J, Howell EA, McLaughlin MA, Stroustrup A, Sundquist K. Pre-term delivery and risk of ischemic heart disease in women. *J Am Coll Cardiol.* 2020;76(1):57-67. doi:10.1016/j.jacc.2020.04.072

161. Lau ES, O'Donoghue ML, Hamilton MA, Goldhaber SZ. Women and heart attacks. *Circulation.* 2016;133(10):e428-e429. doi:10.1161/CIRCULATIONAHA.115.018973

162. Shieh Y, Tice JA. Medications for primary prevention of breast cancer. *JAMA.* 2020;324(3):291-292. doi:10.1001/jama.2020.9246

163. Cuzick J, Sestak I, Cawthorn S, et al. Tamoxifen for prevention of breast cancer: extended long-term follow-up of the IBIS-I breast cancer prevention trial. *Lancet Oncol.* 2015;16(1):67-75. doi:10.1016/S1470-2045(14)71171-4

164. Minami CA, Freedman RA. Menopausal hormone therapy and long-term breast cancer risk: further data from the Women's Health Initiative Trials. *JAMA.* 2020;324(4):347-349. doi:10.1001/jama.2020.9620

165. Winawer SJ, Fletcher RH, Miller L, et al. Colorectal cancer screening: clinical guidelines and rationale [published correction appears in Gastroenterology 1997 Mar;112(3):1060] [published correction appears in Gastroenterology 1998 Mar;114(3):625]. *Gastroenterology.* 1997;112(2):594-642. doi:10.1053/gast.1997.v112.agast970594

166. World Health Organization, Commission on Social Determinants of vasomotor Health. Closing the gap in a generation: health equity through action on the social determinants of health. https://www.who.int/publications/i/item/WHO-IER-CSDH-08.1

167. Roger VL. Medicine and society: social determinants of health and cardiovascular disease. *Eur Heart J.* 2020;41(11):1179-1181. doi:10.1093/eurheartj/ehaa134

168. Tikkanen RS, Schneider EC. Social spending to improve population health - Does the United States spend as wisely as other countries?. *N Engl J Med.* 2020;382(10):885-887. doi:10.1056/NEJMp1916585

169. Schultz WM, Kelli HM, Lisko JC, et al. Socioeconomic status and cardiovascular outcomes: challenges and interventions. *Circulation.* 2018;137(20):2166-2178. doi:10.1161/CIRCULATIONAHA.117.029652

170. Lüscher TF. Towards individualized lifetime risk: combining classical and non-classical factors. *Eur Heart J.* 2020;41(11):1143-1147. doi:10.1093/eurheartj/ehaa155

171. Evans MK. Health equity—Are we finally on the edge of a New Frontier? *N Engl J Med* 2020;383(11):997-999. doi: 10.1056/NEJMp2005944

172. Morrissey M. The state of American retirement savings. Economic Policy Institute, Washington D.C. Published online December 10, 2019. http://epi.org/136219.

173. Koop CE, Lundberg GB. Violence in America: a public health emergency. Time to bite the bullet back [published correction appears in *JAMA* 1992 Dec 2;268(21):3074] [published correction appears in *JAMA* 1994 May 11;271(18):1404]. *JAMA.* 1992;267(22):3075-3076.

174. Kaufman EJ, Wiebe DJ, Xiong RA, et al. Epidemiologic trends in fatal and nonfatal firearm injuries in the US, 2009-2017. *JAMA Intern Med.* 2021;181(2):237-44. doi: 10/1001jamainternmed.2020.6696

175. Grinshteyn E, Hemenway D. Violent death rates: The US compared with other high-income OECD countries, 2010. *Am J Med.* 2016;129(3):266-273. doi:10.1016/j.amjmed.2015.10.025

176. Boockvar KS, Meier DE. Palliative care for frail older adults: "there are things I can't do anymore that I wish I could . . . ". *JAMA.* 2006;296(18):2245-2253. doi:10.1001/jama.296.18.2245

177. Ofori-Asenso R, Chin KL, Mazidi M, et al. Global incidence of frailty and prefrailty among community-dwelling older adults: a systematic review and meta-analysis. *JAMA Netw Open.* 2019;2(8):e198398. Published 2019 Aug 2. doi:10.1001/jamanetworkopen.2019.8398

178. Gwyther H, Shaw R, Jaime Dauden EA, et al. Understanding frailty: a qualitative study of European healthcare policy-makers' approaches to frailty screening and management [published correction appears in *BMJ Open.* 2018 Mar 8;8(3):e018653corr1]. *BMJ Open.* 2018;8(1):e018653. Published 2018 Jan 13. doi:10.1136/bmjopen-2017-018653

179. Lynn J. Reliable and sustainable comprehensive care for frail elderly people. *JAMA.* 2013;310(18):1935-1936. doi:10.1001/jama.2013.281923

180. Visit MediCaring.org for helpful information about elder issues.

181. GBD 2017 US Neurological Disorders Collaborators. Burden on neurological disorders across the US from 1990-2017. A Global Burden of Disease study. *JAMA Neurol.* 2021;78(2):165-176. doi: 10.1001/jamaneurol.2020.4152

182. Holt-Lunstad J, Smith TB, Layton JB. Social relationships and mortality risk: a meta-analytic review. *PLoS Med.* 2010;7(7):e1000316. Published 2010 Jul 27. doi:10.1371/journal.pmed.1000316

183. Gottman J. Here's how healthy couples survive. *The Washington Post.* March 25, 2020. https://www.washingtonpost.com/opinions/2020/03/25/lock down-with-your-partner-heres-how-healthy-couples-survive/

Index

Note: page numbers followed by *f* and *t* refer to figures and tables respectively.

Index

Index

family care for elderly, as no longer
    common, 123, 128–29
family history
    and genetic risk factors, 61, 64, 89, 94,
        98, 113–14, 116
    importance of knowing, 61, 64, 113,
        115
    influence on diet, 25–26
    keeping document with information on,
        benefits of, 85–86, 105
    of neurological disorders, discussing
        with doctor, 127
    and vascular aging, 94*f*
financial crisis of 2007-2008
    and job loss in older men, 47
    and retirement savings, 121, 122*f*
finasteride (Proscar), 82
fitness, and personal reserve, 68
Formative years life period (age 20 to 50),
    9, 10*f*
    balance of prevention, surveillance and
        wellness in, 58*f*
    comorbidities acquired in, importance of
        understanding, 85, 103–5
    difficulty of mitigating damage done in,
        120
    factors affecting health in, 10*f*, 13
    gum (gingivae) recession in, 92–93
    and models of masculinity, 86
    and retirement planning, 14
    surveillance by parents in, 55
frailty
    as acquired risk factor, 62*t*, 104*t*
    age-related changes leading to, 125
    cognitive decline and, 126
    definition of, 125, *126*
    Mediterranean diet and, 65
    prevalence of, 126
    as risk factor, 125
    and safety and security, 125–26
    treatment for, 126
Framingham Heart Study, 20, 55

gastroesophageal reflux (GERD), aging
    and, 87
gay and lesbian community, 131–32

genetic factors in health, 10, 61–64
    breast cancer and, 104*t*, 115
    common genetic diseases, 62*t*, 104*t*
    effect on aging, 62, 64
    and family's health history, importance
        of knowing, 61, 64
    as percentage of health risk, 61
    and vascular aging, 94*f*
GERD. *See* gastroesophageal reflux
    (GERD)
gingivae (gum) recession, in men, with
    aging, 92–93
GI sphincters, effects of aging on, 87–88
glaucoma, Medicare coverage of screenings
    for, 108*t*
Global Burden of Disease study, 66, 126
global planning, need for, 135
Great Depression, and dietary habits,
    25–26
gum (gingivae) recession, in men, with
    aging, 92–93
gun violence
    deaths in 2013 *vs.* 2017, 101*f*
    medical community's current focus on,
        100–101, 118
    as threat to elderly safety and security,
        124
    in US *vs.* other developed countries, 124

hair
    loss and/or change in texture, in men, 91
    whitening of, 91
healing
    reduced blood flow to extremities and,
        92, 111
    skin thinness with aging and, 92, 111
health
    factors affecting, 7, 9, 10*f*
    magnified impact of earlier events, 17–19
    and personal reserve, 68
    preciousness of, 17
    preventive health and medical care and, 7
    pyramid of, 7, 15, 31, 45*f*, 58
    See also genetic factors in health; social
        determinants of health/disease;
        wellness

hemoglobin count, and anemia, 90–91
hepatitis
    history of, as comorbidity, 18*t*
    Medicare coverage of screenings for, 108*t*
herbal remedies
    belief in, as acquired risk factor, 104*t*
    and unintentional injuries in women, 116
high blood pressure. *See* hypertension
high-sensitive CRP (hsCRP), monitoring of, 95, 114
Hispanics
    and COVID-19, unequal treatment during, 120
    life expectancy, recent decline in, 95
    women, and menopausal hot flashes, 106
HIV
    Medicare coverage of screenings for, 108*t*
    and vascular aging, 94*f*
hormonal system
    body mechanisms regulating, 76
    changes with age, 125
hormonal therapies, and breast cancer, 112
"hospitalists," effects on health care, 34, 35–37
hot flashes. *See* menopause, hot flashes in
hsCRP (high-sensitive CRP), monitoring of, 95, 114
Hutchinson-Gilford progeria syndrome, and vascular aging, 94*f*
hyperlipidemia (high cholesterol or triglycerides)
    as genetic risk factor, 62*t*, 104*t*
    health effects of, 18*t*
    Mediterranean diet and, 67
    research on, 20
    as risk factor for cardiovascular disease, 113
    as silent comorbidity, 18*t*, 21, 22–24, 22*f*
hypertension
    age of onset, and risk of cardiovascular disease, 28–29
    effects on heart muscle, 114
    exercise and, 68, 72*f*
    as genetic risk factor, 62*t*, 104*t*
    health effects of, 18*t*, 26

Mediterranean diet and, 66
orthostatic, and falls, 101
poor understanding of, in medical era of 1930–1960, 26–28, 28*f*
research on, 20
as risk factor for cardiovascular disease, 113
silent comorbidities leading to, 18*t*
as silent comorbidity, 18*t*, 21, 22–24, 22*f*
hypothalamus, master clock in, 76, 78

Ikaria (Greece), 73, 128
immunity, and personal reserve, 68
income inequality
    and difficulty of attaining economic peace of mind, 121
    and families' need for two workers, 128
    and low health literacy of low-income persons, 6
    and reduced lifestyle of many in retirement, 122–23
    and risk from COVID-19, 44
    and safety and security of elderly, 124
inflammation
    and anemia, 90–91
    and cardiovascular disease risk, 18*t*, 95
    chronic disease and, 125
    diet and, 44
    of gums (gingivitis), 93
    health effects of, 90–91, 95
    high sensitivity CRP as measure of, 95
    inflammatory cardiovascular biomarkers, diet and, 66, 66*f*
    insomnia and, 75
influenza
    annual vaccine, benefits of, 80–81
    as leading cause of death in US, 60*t*
informed consent of patients, and shared healthcare decision making, 50
injuries, unintentional
    as leading cause of death in US, 59, 60*t*
    See also falls; men, unintentional injuries in; sports injuries; women, unintentional injuries in
insomnia, 74–75

rectal cancer. *See* colon/rectal cancer
regularity
    adaptive types of, 76
    body clocks and, 76–77
    in bowel function, 75–76, 78
    circadian rhythm and, 74, 76
    effect of environment on, 73
    impaired personal reserve and, 77–78
    non-adaptive types of, 76
remdesivir, and COVID-19, 82
residence, region of, and life expectancy, 25
respiratory disease, chronic
    efforts to reduce, 21
    as leading cause of death, 21, 59, 60*t*
retirement
    expectations for, in American culture, 13
    reduced lifestyle of many in, 122–23
    savings for
        as inadequate for most of population, 14, 121–22, 122*f*
        by level of education, 123*f*
        as part of US culture, 13–14
rheumatoid arthritis, and vascular aging, 94*f*
risk factors. *See* health risk factors
Roosevelt, Franklin D., hypertension contributing to death of, 26–28, 28*f*

safety and security, 124–27
    and cognitive decline, 126–27
    health crises and, 124–25
    income inequality and, 124
    onset of frailty and, 125–26
    organizations formed to address, 126
    physical vulnerability of elderly and, 124
    threat of crime and violence and, 124
SARS-coronavirus-2. *See* COVID-19
secondary smoke
    health effects of, 11, 18*t*
    as silent comorbidity, 18*t*, 22*f*
Second Woman's Health Initiative, 106
sedentary lifestyle
    and cancer risk, 98
    and cardiovascular disease risk, 95
    health effects of, 18*t*
    as health risk factor, 21, 62*t*, 104*t*

increase in, 69
    and osteoporosis, 107
    and risk of menopausal hot flashes, 106
    as silent comorbidity, 18*t*, 22*f*, 69
self-harm, as leading cause of death in US, 60*t*
    See also suicide
sexual dysfunction, cardiovascular disease and, 94
sexual intercourse, pain for women in, 111, 112
sexually transmitted diseases, Medicare coverage of screenings for, 108*t*
shared decision-making in health care, 49–51
Sheldon, William, 62–64
shelter, inadequate, health effects of, 57
shingles vaccine (Shingrix), benefits of, 80–81
shivering, regulation of, 77
shots, Medicare coverage for, 108*t*
skin cancer, incidence, by year and gender, 99*f*
skin thinness
    in men, 91–92
    in women, 111
sleep, 73–75
    afternoon naps, 74
    changes in, with aging, 74
    and circadian rhythm, 74
    disturbances and irregularities, as risk factor, 73–75
    insomnia, 74–75
    menopausal hot flashes and, 106
    normal, health benefits of, 75
    optimal amount of, 73
    and vascular aging, 94*f*
sleep apnea
    exercise and, 68
    health effects of, 18*t*, 23, 73, 90
    obesity and, 73
    obstructive *vs.* central type, 73
    as silent comorbidity, 18*t*, 22*f*
smart phones
    as health care tool, 135–36
    and wearable health care technologies, 44

Permissions

Figure 10 on p. 66 reprinted by permission from Li J, Lee DH, Hu J, et al. Dietary Inflammatory Potential and Risk of Cardiovascular Disease Among Men and Women in the U.S. (Central Illustration). *J Am Coll Cardiol.* 2020;76(19):2181-2193. https://www.sciencedirect.com/science/article/pii/S0735109720371904?via%3Dihub

Figure 15 (top) on p. 96 reprinted by permission from Libby P, Ridker PM, Maseri A. Inflammation and atherosclerosis. (Fig. 1) *Circulation.* 2002;105(9):1135-1143. https://www.ahajournals.org/doi/10.1161/hc0902.104353

Figure 15 (bottom) reprinted by permission from Naghavi M, Libby P, Falk E, et al. From vulnerable plaque to vulnerable patient: a call for new definitions and risk assessment strategies: Part I. (Fig. 2) *Circulation.* 2003;108(14):1664-1672. https://www.ahajournals.org/doi/10.1161/01.CIR.0000087480.94275.97